Leadership

The Key to the Professionalization of Nursing

Leadership

The Key to the Professionalization of Nursing

Linda Anne Bernhard, RN, MS
Assistant Professor
Rush University

Practitioner/Teacher
Rush-Presbyterian-St. Luke's Medical Center
Chicago, Illinois

Michelle Walsh, RN, MS
Doctoral Student
University of Illinois at the Medical Center
Chicago, Illinois

McGraw-Hill Book Company

New York St. Louis San Francisco Auckland Bogotá Guatemala Hamburg
Johannesburg Lisbon London Madrid Mexico Montreal New Delhi
Panama Paris San Juan São Paulo Singapore Sydney Tokyo Toronto

This book was set in Press Roman by Allen Wayne Technical Corp.
The editor was Laura A. Dysart;
the production supervisor was Nancy Parisotti;
the cover was designed by Charles A. Carson.

LEADERSHIP: THE KEY TO THE PROFESSIONALIZATION OF NURSING

Library of Congress Cataloging in Publication Data

Bernhard, Linda A
    Leadership: the key to the professionalization
of nursing.

    Bibliography: p.
    Includes index.
    1. Nursing service administration. 2. Leadership.
I. Walsh, Michelle, joint author. II. Title.
RT89.B45   610.73'06'9   80-21957
ISBN 0-07-004936-X

To our grandmothers
Marie E. Darnell
and
Cecile C. Hagerty

Contents

Preface

Leadership in nursing is a topic of great concern among nursing educators and nursing service personnel. Nursing must have leaders to become professionalized. Since leadership can be learned, we believe that nurses should be educated to become leaders. The purpose of this book then is to assist in teaching nurses to become leaders and to promote the professionalization of nursing.

The book is organized according to concepts essential to the practice of nursing leadership. Each chapter may be considered as a unit which encompasses the theoretical basis of the concept and its application to nursing. Thus, the chapters could be read in any order. However, there was a conscious effort to sequence the chapters in an order which allows the reader to consider first the components of leadership and then the specific strategies used by nurse-leaders.

An analysis of the professionalization of nursing is presented in the first chapter. From this analysis, the need for nurse-leaders and a theory of leadership becomes clear.

Nursing leadership is a multidimensional process which depends upon the relationship between the nurse-leader and a group, the setting or organization in which the interaction occurs, and the theory of leadership chosen by the nurse-leader. These three components are considered as separate entities in Chapters 2, 3, and 4. Chapter 5 explores the three components as a unified whole that provides direction to the nurse-leader.

A variety of strategies can be used in nursing leadership to enhance the nurse-leader's effectiveness. These strategies—organizing, teaching-learning, decision making, changing, managing conflict, and evaluating—are considered in Chapters 6 through 11.

The epilogue suggests that the professionalization of nursing is possible, and will occur when nurse-leaders actualize nursing leadership. An attempt has been made to stimulate nurse-leaders to ask questions about their practice, and to continue to question the extent of the professionalization of nursing.

Leadership: The Key to the Professionalization of Nursing is intended primarily for use as a textbook in all baccalaureate nursing programs—both generic and RN/BSN completion. It may be used in leadership courses, or in other courses where leadership and other management concepts are studied. Educators and students in other types of nursing programs may find the book a useful resource for discussion of issues related to professional nursing.

The book will be helpful also to in-service educators and staff development personnel for orienting new graduates to leadership roles within their institutions. In addition, the book could be used as a reference for all staff nurses who wish to function more effectively in their roles as nurse-leaders.

We would like to acknowledge our families, friends, and colleagues who supported us in this endeavor.

Linda Anne Bernhard
Michelle Walsh

Chapter 1

The Professionalization of Nursing

The conflict over whether or not nursing is a profession has existed for many years and it continues today. Before this conflict can be resolved conclusively, an acceptable definition of "profession" must be found.

Flexner's classic definition of profession is often used. Flexner identified six criteria that a work group must possess to acquire professional status. These are: (1) the activities of the work group must be intellectual; (2) the activities, because they are based on knowledge, can be learned; (3) the work activities must be practical, as opposed to academic or theoretical; (4) the profession must have teachable techniques, which are the work of professional education; (5) there must be a strong internal organization of members of the work group; and (6) altruism, a desire to provide for the good of society, must be the workers' motivating force (Flexner, 1915).

Since Flexner evolved these criteria, numerous authors have attempted to rewrite, add to, or subtract from them. A composite list of criteria for today would include the existence of a body of knowledge unique to that work group, which would be established through research and logical scientific analysis. In addition, an individual must be able to acquire that body of knowledge—usually through a long period of study—and he or she should be taught by existing members of the work group. Another criterion would be the presence of a committed group of members who have and enforce a code of ethics.

The criteria established to define a profession have been termed idealistic, and even unrealistic. Since it is virtually impossible for every member of a profession to fulfill every criterion exactly, no work group could ever truly be a "profession" (Becker, 1962; Vollmer & Mills, 1966). However, most work groups, including nursing, strive to reach that ideal, largely because of the prestige and status that being a profession has brought to such groups as medicine and law.

Consequently, the idea of professionalization has developed. *Professionalization* is a dynamic process through which occupations change certain crucial characteristics in the direction of a profession (Vollmer & Mills, 1966, pp. vii–viii).

A specific sequence of steps in the professionalization process has been identified by Caplow (1954). First, a professional association with explicit membership criteria is formed. Next, the name of the work group is changed in order to reduce identification with the old occupation and to monopolize a new title and domain. Then a code of ethics is established. Finally, political agitation takes place to establish legal codes for licensing and practice. Concurrently with these activities, educational facilities are developed, under the direct or indirect control of the professional association (Caplow, 1954, pp. 139–140).

It is helpful to conceptualize the progress toward the professionalization as a continuum on which the left end is occupation, or nonprofession, and the right end is profession.

Occupation (O)————————————————(P) Profession

THE OCCUPATION-PROFESSION CONTINUUM MODEL

Pavalko (1971), a sociologist, has established a continuum model of professionalization that can be used by any prospective profession to determine how professionalized it is. Pavalko includes eight categories, or criteria, and the work group is measured against each of them. He states that any other criteria which an individual may consider more representative of professional status can be subsumed within the eight (Pavalko, 1971, p. 17). Pavalko's criteria will be presented below and applied to the present situation of nursing.

Theory

The first category is the presence of theory, or intellectual technique; the work group is judged on the extent to which its work is based on a systematic body of theory and abstract knowledge (Pavalko, 1971, p. 18). The greater the body of knowledge, the more professional is the group.

Systematic theory comes only through research, and research in nursing is relatively new. Most initial "nursing research" centered around *nurses*, and was carried out by social scientists as early as the 1930s. *Nursing Research* journal was established in 1952 with the expressed purpose of informing members of the nursing profession and other professions about the results of scientific studies in nursing, and of stimulating research in nursing. This publication was successful in encouraging nurses to carry out and publish research. Research findings are now also being published in other nursing journals, and additional journals with the purpose of communicating nursing research have been developed.

Since 1970, the American Nurses' Association (ANA) has become very involved in research through the Commission on Nursing Research, which was established to address the research concerns of the profession. In 1971, the Council of Nurse Researchers was formed to address the special concerns of those researchers. Finally, nursing research is now focusing on the clinical practice of *nursing;* thus, scientific bases for nursing practice are being established.

Because research in nursing, and especially in clinical practice, is so new, the theory base of nursing is just being developed. With regard to theory, nursing can therefore be considered to be about midway along the occupation-profession continuum.

Criterion 1:   O ————————●———————— P

Relevance to Basic Social Values

The second category is the relevance to basic social values of the work performed (Pavalko, 1971, p. 18). What this means is that the professions tend to justify their existence by identifying themselves with abstract values on which there is general societal consensus, for example, life, liberty, and the pursuit of happiness. Occupations do not need such a justification to exist and they may not be relevant to social values. This category could also be called "application to crucial problems of society" or "matters of great urgency and significance" (McGlothlin 1964, p. 4).

Nursing, like medicine, fulfills this criterion because of its concern for the individual's well-being. Nursing deals with people at all levels of health, from birth through death.[1]

Nursing may be placed at the right end of the continuum because of its obvious relationship to many social values and concerns.

Criterion 2:   O ———————————————————●P

Training or Educational Period

The training (or educational) period, Pavalko's third category, has four subdimensions (Pavalko, 1971, p. 19). The amount or length of education, the degree of specialization involved, the use of symbolic and ideational processes, and the actual content are all important elements in education.

In general, the professional end of the continuum is characterized by a long period of education, with a high degree of specialization and a strong emphasis on the ability to manipulate ideas and symbols as well as things. In addition to the knowledge and skills necessary for the profession, the content of professional education includes a

---

[1] Health is viewed by these authors as including illness. A person always has a health status, i.e., the level of health at the present time, and a health potential, i.e., the highest level of health possible for that individual. We believe that baccalaureate nursing students should be focusing on health—its promotion, maintenance, and restoration. This is not to deny that illness exists, but rather to emphasize that the nurse should focus, not on illness, but on restoring the person's health.

specific set of values, norms, and roles that each member of the profession is expected to develop. These values, norms, and roles characterize the "professional subculture," or the unique qualities that distinguish that group of workers from all other groups.

For each subdimension the position on the occupational end of the continuum may vary. For example, occupational education usually takes a short time—from a few weeks to a few months—in the case of a ward secretary. It may, however, take two or more years, as in the case of a rehabilitation assistant, or there may be no educational requirement, as in the case of a playroom supervisor on a pediatrics unit.

Florence Nightingale, the founder of modern nursing, envisioned an education for nurses which would include both theory and practice (Nutting & Dock, 1907, p. 201). Unfortunately, because nursing schools developed in hospitals in the United States, and because the need for nurses was so great, nursing education became limited to the teaching of specific techniques with little theory presented.

Over the years, some nurses have worked to make nursing education conform more closely to Florence Nightingale's ideal, that is, to include both theory and practice. Although progress has been slow, nursing education is gradually moving out of service institutions (hospitals) and into educational institutions (colleges and universities).

In 1965, the ANA published a position paper which stated that nursing education should take place in institutions of higher education, and that the baccalaureate degree should be the minimum preparation for professional nursing. However, in 1975, when the New York State Nurses' Association voted to recommend legislation that would require a baccalaureate degree for licensure as a professional nurse by 1985 (20 years *after* the position paper), many nurses were upset. Nurses across the country are still debating the so-called "entry into professional practice" issue. Once emotions are eliminated, the issue can be reduced to one of theory and practice.

The length of education for the registered nurse varies greatly, from 2 years for the associate degree to 4 or 5 years for the baccalaureate degree. In the past, initial degrees in nursing were also awarded at the master's level. The newest initial degree in nursing is the *nursing doctorate* (ND) which was initiated as a new program at Frances Payne Bolton School of Nursing, Case Western Reserve University, in 1979. The nursing doctorate is built upon the baccalaureate degree and will take 3 years to complete.

Graduate education in nursing also varies greatly. Master's degree programs vary from 1 to 2 years and may result in master of science (MS), master of arts (MA), master of science in nursing (MSN), or master of nursing (MN) degrees. Doctoral programs lead to doctor of nursing science (DNS), doctor of science in nursing (DSN), and doctor of philosophy (Ph.D) degrees, with differing expectations in each type of program.

Nursing is becoming more and more specialized, and nurses are taught many special skills. The medical model specialties of medical-surgical nursing, pediatric nursing, obstetric nursing, and psychiatric nursing are being further divided into such subspecialties as critical care nursing, neonatal nursing, and gerontological nursing. In addition there is public, or community health nursing, which is also rapidly developing subspecialties. Other specialty skills, such as physical assessment, are now being incorporated into most nursing educational programs.

As nursing moves into the mainstream of education, it is focusing more on theory and emphasizing scientific rationale rather than just techniques of care. College-based education also stresses a broad general education for nurses so that a better understanding of human beings and society is developed. A heavy emphasis has always been placed on the *professional socialization* (development of the identity and culture of the profession) (Pavalko, 1971, p. 82) of nursing students, and this must continue.

Nursing falls far short of being a profession with regard to the educational criterion because of the great variability in the length and type of nursing education programs. However, because more theory and specialized content are being taught, and because the professional subculture maintains its strength, nursing may be placed a little more than halfway across the occupation-profession continuum.

Criterion 3:   O ————————————●———————— P

Motivation

Motivation for work is the fourth category in the model (Pavalko, 1971, p. 20). The motivation of a particular individual is difficult to evaluate and is not what Pavalko was referring to in this category. Rather, motivation means the extent to which the work group emphasizes the ideal of service to the public, and not merely service to its own interests, as its primary goal. A profession is expected to have a higher interest in serving the public and also in making its goals and motivation known.

Nursing developed as a service to society. Nurses have nearly always been considered altruistic and nurturant, and today they still identify publicly their desire to help and serve people.

In one study, "thousands" of young women who had chosen nursing as a career were asked why they made that choice. Almost all said they wanted to "help those in need of help" (Hampton, 1972, p. 2). During 1974 and 1975, 114 persons who had completed one baccalaureate degree and were entering nursing were studied. When asked why they chose nursing, "fully a third" said the reason was their interest in people and desire to help others (Smith, 1976, p. 89).

Nurses indicate their desire for service to persons when they become involved with events, organizations, and issues in society and identify themselves as nurses. Examples include Wilma Scott Heide, former president of the National Organization for Women; Susan D. Rogers and Connie Engel, the first women pilots to graduate from the United States Air Force; and Lillian Carter, former executive director of the Georgia Nurses' Association. Numerous other nurses volunteer their time and energy to such organizations as the Red Cross, American Cancer Society, and crisis intervention centers.

Because of its continuing goal of service and its history of altruism, nursing may be placed at the right end of the occupation-profession continuum.

Criterion 4:   O ———————————————————●P

Autonomy

A fifth category is autonomy, which means the freedom of the work group to regulate and control its own work behavior (Pavalko, 1971, p. 22). Usually work groups at the occupation end of the continuum are subject to many external controls, controls that come from outside or above the group. Work groups at the profession end of the continuum have more self-regulation, or internal controls, which are established through consensus by the members in the group.

Individuals who are employed by someone else are under the (external) control of their employer, i.e., they must do what the employer wants. Individuals who own their own business, or who jointly own businesses, have their own rules or governance plan (i.e., internal controls).

In terms of autonomy, nursing has many positive and some negative aspects. The autonomy of the profession as a whole is increasing because many state nurse practice acts are being revised to allow nurses a broader scope of practice, particularly in the areas of diagnosis[2] and treatment of patient problems. This change is a result of the hard work of many nurses who want to increase internal controls.

In 1967, the ANA Divisions of Practice began to write standards for nursing practice. The first standards, published in 1973, were the *Standards of Nursing Practice* (ANA, 1973). These standards serve as a guide for all nursing practice. Also in 1973, standards were published for two of the specialty groups. In 1980, there are at least 17 different sets of standards, with some of them being revised and new ones being written. It is by using these standards that greater and stronger internal controls of nursing, by nurses, can be maintained.

Two major problems exist with regard to the autonomy of nursing. First, most nurses are employees of institutions, and second, whether they are employed or not, many nurses still believe in the authority of the physician and feel subservient to the physician, or at least pretend that they do (McGee & Martin, 1978, p. 50).

Nurses have had difficulty establishing and maintaining *peer* controls, because in the past they were mainly employees who were evaluated by *supervisors*. Peers have had little power or control over each other because of the lack of rewards and punishments. However, by using their nursing standards, nurses are establishing peer review, and are openly evaluating one another.

Nurses have begun to bargain collectively, often through state nurses' associations, and bargaining has been successful in many cases: working hours and conditions have improved, and salaries and fringe benefits have increased.

The power of physicians over nurses still exists, since many nurses, physicians, and the society at large still consider nurses as something less than, and under the control of, physicians (Ehrenreich & Ehrenreich, 1975, p. 48). However, some nurses now see their roles as overlapping with physicians' roles (Trinosky, 1979, p. 41), and they are becoming more assertive in dealing with physicians. Furthermore, as medicine and nursing become more specialized, physicians are beginning to give up some of their power to nurses whom they trust. It must also be remembered that, of the many functions nurses perform, only one is a dependent function—that of carrying out the physician's orders; for the remainder, nurses function independently or interdependently with other health team members (Lesnik & Anderson, 1955, p. 277).

---

[2] That is, nursing, not medical, diagnosis and treatment. Nursing diagnosis is a descriptive interpretation of all the data collected regarding the client's problems and/or needs. See F. L. Bower. *The process of planning nursing care*. St. Louis: Mosby, 1977, p. 13.

Although nursing has many problems in seeking autonomy, it also has many strengths. Because of its strengths, nursing may be placed on the right half of the continuum.

Criterion 5:   O ——————————————●————— P

Sense of Commitment

The sixth category is the sense of commitment the members have toward their work (Pavalko, 1971, p. 23). At the profession end of the continuum, work is viewed as a lifetime, or at least long-term, commitment. At the occupation end, this dedication is apt to be absent, and movement into and out of an occupation is common.

Commitment to the profession of nursing has traditionally been very low and nursing has experienced a drastic dropout rate. In the past, most nurses were women who, though initially interested in nursing and service to people, often married and left nursing to raise families. Very few returned to nursing, even when their children were grown.

Fortunately, this situation is changing. Married women are seeing roles for themselves in addition to those of wife and mother. Women today are generally more career-oriented than in the past, and more women are managing their homes *and* their nursing careers. Some nurses still drop out, but tend to return to nursing when their youngest child is in school. Others work part-time throughout the child-rearing period. It is essential that this increase in commitment continue because no profession can afford to lose a majority of the persons it has educated.

Another problem regarding commitment has been identified by Kramer (1974). Many new graduates with a strong commitment to nursing are shocked to find that the professional ideals and values developed in school are neither practiced nor rewarded in the work setting (p. viii). Without help and guidance through this "reality shock," some nurses leave nursing.[3]

Although change is occurring, nursing can be placed no further than midway on the occupation-profession continuum because there are still a great many persons who have been educated as nurses who are not working, and there are still many nurses who drop out.[4]

Criterion 6:   O ——————————●——————————— P

Sense of Community

The seventh category (Pavalko, 1971, p. 24), sense of community, means the degree to which members of the work group share a common identity and destiny and possess a

---

[3] For a complete understanding of the reality shock phenomenon, read M. Kramer. *Reality shock: Why nurses leave nursing.* St. Louis: Mosby, 1974; for an understanding of how to help the reality shock victim, read M. Kramer & C. E. Schmalenberg. *Path to biculturalism.* Wakefield, Mass.: Contemporary Publishing, 1977.

[4] Hard data that documents these issues is very limited. Studies to determine why nurses drop out and the exact number who do are desperately needed.

distinctive subculture. This subculture significantly influences the work behavior and even the nonwork behaviors of group members. The sense of community is apt to be low at the occupation end of the continuum, high at the profession end.

Nursing has a distinctive subculture, one which was traditionally encouraged with the uniform, cap, and pin. Use of these symbols is changing as many nurses come to believe that it is not what they wear that makes them nurses; however, there is still a strong feeling of identity among nurses.

Nursing's professional organization is the American Nurses' Association, founded in 1897 as the National Associated Alumnae of the United States and Canada.[5] The organization is strong and has professional lobbyists who are able to exert influence on legislation affecting nursing and the health and welfare of the public.

As strong as the ANA is, however, membership in the organization is low.[6] Several reasons may account for this. One is that numerous nursing specialty organizations exist, such as the American Association of Critical-Care Nurses (AACN) and the Association of Operating Room Nurses (AORN), which tend to attract members away from ANA. This is because some nurses feel a greater sense of community with nurses who share their problems.[7] Although some of these organizations encourage membership in ANA as well as in the specialty group, many of them do not, and many individuals who belong to specialty organizations do not join ANA whether or not the organization encourages them to belong.

A second reason for ANA's low membership may be the existence of the National League for Nursing (NLN), an organization whose goal is "helping to meet the nursing needs of the people," and one which allows nonnurses to belong. This organization is large and, like ANA, exerts a great deal of power; there have, however, been many conflicts between the two associations, and some nurses have chosen to give their allegiance to just one of the two.

Another factor which may influence the membership in ANA is that all registered nurses—those in direct clinical practice, as well as administrators, educators, and researchers—are permitted to join. These different members have different needs, concerns, and educational preparation. Belonging to the same organization provides a positive sense of community, but it can also cause problems if some members feel that their needs and concerns are unheard or unmet.

A fairly recent problem related to ANA membership stems from its economic and general welfare program, and its commitment to collective bargaining for its members. With the amendments to the Taft-Hartley Act in 1974, the ANA can be considered a

[5] Part of the professional socialization of nurses has been an emphasis on the social and professional relationships among nurses. Alumni associations have been and still are very strong organizations of nurses.

[6] The most recent figures obtainable from the ANA reflect data collected in September 1977. At that time there were about 1.4 million registered nurses in the United States, and only 191,000 were members of ANA—less than 14 percent.

[7] That is, problems of a day-to-day clinical practice nature, as opposed to the general problems of the profession, which are the primary concern of the ANA.

labor union. As a result, membership in ANA has become a problem for "supervisory" nurses, who are forced into a conflict of interest by being a member both of management *and* of a labor union. Many nurses in nursing service administration have therefore cancelled their memberships in ANA to avoid this conflict.

Other reasons why nurses may not join the professional organization include cost of dues, lack of time, a feeling of no personal benefit from membership, and general apathy. The fact that these feelings still exist and are verbalized indicates that the sense of community in nursing needs to be further developed.

The problems related to a sense of community seem to be problems of individual nurses. As a group, nurses feel unity and pride. Therefore, in spite of the problems, nursing can be placed near the right end of the continuum.

Criterion 7:　　O ————————————————●—— P

Code of Ethics

The final category in Pavalko's model is the existence of a code of ethics (Pavalko, 1971, p. 25). At the occupation end of the continuum the code is apt to be undeveloped, perhaps unwritten, and to have few relationships spelled out. The further right a group moves on the continuum, the more formal is the code. The complexity of the code, the number of behaviors and relationships described, and the enforceability of the code usually increase as a work group becomes more professionalized.

The ANA has had a written code of ethics since 1950, 3 years before the International Council of Nurses published its code. The code has been revised several times and each revision has improved the code and made it more explicit. The present code, as revised in 1976, includes an explanation for each statement (ANA, 1976). Included in the code are such things as how the nurse should function with clients and what the nurse should do for the profession. The ANA, through its state organizations, maintains the power to enforce the code.[8]

Because nursing has a well-written code of ethics with a large number of behaviors and relationships spelled out, and because the code is enforced through the professional organization, nursing may be considered to be at the right end of the occupation-profession continuum.

Criterion 8:　　O ——————————————————●P

If one places the eight categories together, as shown in Figure 1-1, it is obvious that nursing has significant lags in the professionalization process. The unshaded portion of the figure shows the areas in which nursing must place its greatest efforts. Areas needing most work are theory, education, autonomy, and commitment.

---

[8] Every nurse should keep a copy of the code for personal use. The code is available from the ANA or from state nurses' associations for a minimal fee.

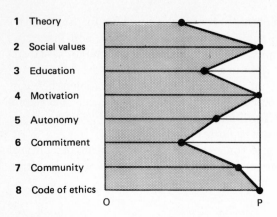

Figure 1-1   Extent of the professionalization of nursing.   (O = occupation, P = profession)

SUMMARY

Achievement of true professional status is a valid goal for nursing, and gains are being made, but nurse-leaders must work diligently to continue the process. Unfortunately, until recently, nursing expected nurses to become leaders without formal education or training in leadership, and to work for nursing just because they were nurses. It is now realized that nurses need knowledge, skills, and tools in order to exert leadership and thus cope with the problems inherent in the process of professionalization.

Nursing exists to serve the patient and society, and the professionalization of nursing will ultimately help society. Leadership is a process which can be used in any situation, simple or complex, to further professionalize nursing. As nurses utilize leadership and recognize the power they can achieve, they will see that leadership is indeed the key to the professionalization of nursing.

REFERENCES

American Nurses' Association. *Code for nurses with interpretive statements.* Kansas City, 1976.

American Nurses' Association. *Standards of nursing practice.* Kansas City, 1973.

Becker, H. S. The nature of a profession. In N. B. Henry (Ed.), *Education for the professions.* Chicago: University of Chicago Press, 1962.

Caplow, T. *The sociology of work.* Minneapolis: University of Minnesota Press, 1954.

Ehrenreich, B., & Ehrenreich, J. H. Hospital workers: Class conflicts in the making. *International Journal of Health Services*, 1975, *5*, 43–51.

Flexner, A. Is social work a profession? *Proceedings of the National Conference of Charities and Correction.* Chicago: Hildman, 1915.

Hampton, P. J. Why they choose nursing. *Journal of Nursing Education*, 1972, *11*(1), 2–7.

Kramer, M. *Reality shock: Why nurses leave nursing.* St. Louis, Mosby, 1974.

Lesnik, M. J., & Anderson, B. E. *Nursing practice and the law.* Philadelphia: Lippincott, 1955.

McGee, A. D., & Martin, W. B. W. The games nurses play. *Canadian Nurse*, 1978, *74*(7), 49–52.

McGlothlin, W. J. *The professional schools.* New York: Center for Applied Research in Education, 1964.

Nutting, M. A., & Dock, L. L. *A history of nursing* (Vol. 2). New York: Putnam, 1907.

Pavalko, R. M. *Sociology of occupations and professions.* Itasca, Ill.: Peacock, 1971.

Smith, R. A. Why college graduates choose nursing. *Nursing Outlook*, 1976, *24*, 88–91.

Trinosky, P. Nurse-doctor dissension still thrives. *Supervisor Nurse*, 1979, *10*(4), 40–43.

Vollmer, H. M., & Mills, D. L. (Eds.). *Professionalization.* Englewood Cliffs, N.J.: Prentice-Hall, 1966.

ADDITIONAL READINGS

American Nurses' Association's first position on education for nursing. *American Journal of Nursing*, 1965, *65*(12), 106–111.

Chaska, N. L. (Ed.). *The nursing profession: Views through the mist.* New York: McGraw-Hill, 1978.

Kellams, S. E. Ideals of a profession: The case of nursing. *Image*, 1977, *9*, 30–31.

McBride, A. et al. Leadership: Problems and possibilities in nursing. *American Journal of Nursing*, 1972, *72*, 1445–1456.

McClure, M. L. The long road to accountability. *Nursing Outlook*, 1978, *26*, 47–50.

McGriff, E. P. The courage for effective leadership in nursing. *Image*, 1976, *8*, 56–60.

NYSNA calls for B.S. degree as basis for nurse licensure by 1985. *American Journal of Nursing*, 1975, *75*, 2109, 2112–2113.

Schirger, M. J. Introspection: A prerequisite for emancipation. *Nursing Forum*, 1978, *17*, 317–328.

Chapter 2

The Leader
and the Group

Leadership is a process which is used to move a group toward goal setting and goal achievement. The leadership process may be used by any person; therefore, any person can theoretically be a leader at any given time. Leadership can also be learned.

Learning about leadership begins with understanding what constitutes a leader and a group. There are three requirements for being a leader: (1) one must have a goal or an idea to which one is strongly committed; (2) one must have a follower to lead; and (3) one must employ the leadership process.

A group is a number of individuals working together to achieve a goal. A group may be a dyad, having only the leader and one member, or it may have any number of members. Each individual member of the group may be termed "follower."

THE LEADER

One may become a leader in two ways. The first way is to be informally chosen or formally elected to the position by members of the group. The members, or followers, have thus recognized and accepted the leader's influence, and have selected him or her to lead them. This has been called *emergent leadership* (Hollander, 1964, p. 6).

The second way is to be appointed or elected to the position by a person or group external to the group to be led. For example, a new head nurse for a nursing unit may be appointed by the hospital administration. The nursing staff on the unit—the group that the new head nurse will lead—may have no voice in the selection. Another example is the assignment of a particular nurse to care for a given patient; the patient (group) has no choice in the appointment of the nurse (leader). This has been called *imposed* or *organizational leadership* (Hollander, 1964, p. 6).

The advantages to emergent leadership are that the followers view the leader as someone who is competent and someone whom they trust and value (Hollander, 1961, p. 38). The imposed leader may have a difficult time being accepted by the group and receiving its support because the group does not know and trust the leader.

Ideally, the emergent leader and the imposed leader is the same person. If the group members have a say in the choice of leader, their choice (emergent) may be the one that the superior authority appoints (imposed).

It is more likely that the imposed leader and the emergent leader will be different persons. There are several reasons why this may happen, such as (1) the group selects an emergent leader, but another is imposed; (2) the imposed leader is incompetent, so an emergent leader is chosen; or (3) the group disagrees with the imposed leader's approach, so an emergent leader is selected.

A problem exists when the imposed and emergent leaders are different persons. In this situation, it is not clear to the group who is in charge, and because of the confusion the group cannot function effectively. Consequently, morale and productivity decrease.

All types of leaders can be classified as having become leaders in one of two ways. It was stated before that a leader must have a group. Either the *leader* (e.g., a religious or political leader) *seeks a group*, or the *group selects the leader*. In both cases these are emergent leaders.

Leaders who seek a group often are ahead of their time, i.e., they have ideas which are viewed as very forward-looking. In nursing, a leader who sought a group was Lillian Wald, the founder of public health nursing. A leader who is selected by a group often is an elected official such as Isabel Hampton Robb, the first president of the American Nurses' Association.

Awareness, assertiveness, accountability, and advocacy are four important attributes for the effective leader. These four attributes are interrelated. Awareness of self and of the group is a prerequisite to assertiveness, and advocacy depends on acting assertively and accounting for one's actions. Each of these attributes will be discussed in detail.

Awareness

Leaders must be very aware of *themselves* and of all their characteristics, so that they are able to assess their effects on the group. There are several specific areas of self-awareness that the leader should analyze.

The first is degree of *maturity*. If maturity is defined as the willingness and ability to do a task (Hersey & Blanchard, 1977, p. 161), the leader must be aware of his or her motivation and knowledge base regarding the task. Motivation is vital to effective leadership. The leader must *want* to be a leader. Being a leader is a large task; it involves the willingness and ability of the leader to accept responsibility, not only for his or her own actions, but also for the actions of the group.

A leader's *ability* will depend on knowledge of the area of responsibility.

Strengths and limitations regarding the topic or problem at hand must be identified. Further, the leader must be willing to work to minimize the limitations, and must be well-informed about resources, both material and human, that can aid both group and leader in their endeavor. A leader cannot feel truly comfortable in the role as leader if he or she does not know a great deal about the subject under consideration.

Since commitment to a goal is one of the requirements for being a leader, continual awareness and assessment of *goals* is necessary. Many things are necessary to achieve goals, among them time, money, and persons. Goals must be sound and realistic.

The leader should be able to set appropriate short-term goals that will ultimately lead to achievement of the overall goal. In addition, the leader must be able to communicate these goals to the followers, and help them set and accomplish goals which will also lead to achievement of the larger goal.

Awareness of *power*—how it is achieved and how it is used—is very important. The leader must first recognize that he or she *has* power. Often power is achieved by virtue of position; it is given by a superior, so that a task can be carried out. Power is also given to the leader by the group; they defer to the leader because he or she is trusted and seen as an expert (Goldstein & Sorcher, 1974, p. 6).

The leader must also be aware of how power is used. It can be used in the traditional and negative sense, which implies getting the group to do what the leader wants them to do; or it can be shared with the group, so that all members have equal participation. The interaction of leader and members helps to establish a group power base which can be directed toward goal achievement.

Careful assessment of a leader's *personality* and how he or she is viewed by others is important. Leaders should be aware of the extent of their self-confidence, enthusiasm, flexibility, creativity, honesty, sincerity, tact, and friendliness, since this awareness will lead to a clearer understanding of how they affect others. Personal appearance is also of concern. Knowledge of assets and liabilities in these areas will help the leader to use self to best advantage in influencing the group.

To relate to group members, the leader utilizes various *communication skills*, and attempts to convey a clear, straightforward message to the group. The leader then looks for a response that will indicate whether the intended message was received. An awareness of both the leader's and the group's verbal and nonverbal communication behaviors is important. Diligent attention is given to receiving the messages from the group. The communication network which is established allows the leader to influence group members.

Another area of self-awareness for the leader to analyze is his or her *endurance*. Endurance refers to physical and emotional limits. An effective leader often functions under a great deal of stress and pressure, and therefore must be aware of how stress is managed.

An important ability for a leader is knowing how to say "no." Often when one becomes a leader, and enjoys being a leader, one takes on more and more responsibilities and may finally become greatly overextended. A person who is overstressed gives, or gains, little. Consequently, the effective leader knows when the limits have been reached, and is able to say "no."

Of course the leader must also be able to say "yes," and take on or seek out other responsibilities if his or her limits have not been reached. Otherwise, one will not stay a leader for long.

In relation to endurance, the leader must also be aware of how he or she deals with success and failure, of how to be gracious in both success and failure, and of how to use both as incentives for future successes. Successes are usually easy to accept, but it takes great skill and perseverance to pick up the pieces after a defeat and go on. The effective leader must be able to continue the work, and to help the group continue.

In addition to being aware of self, the leader must also be aware of the group—both individual members and the group as a whole. Each member's goals, needs, abilities, and values, as well as his or her feelings about belonging to the group, are important in relation to that person's ability to function within the group. An effective leader will assess the member's strengths and limitations, and get to know the member as an individual, so that he or she can assist the person to overcome limitations, work toward potential, and be a productive member of the group.

Knowing each individual well will help the leader to predict the goals, needs, abilities, and values, as well as the strengths, limitations, and potential of the whole group. But, for the group to work effectively, each individual member must fuse into the group. The leader facilitates this fusion by having empathy for each individual member.

Communication among group members is essential for any productive work to occur; therefore, the leader must be aware of the communication patterns within the group. The leader must know which persons participate extensively, which participate minimally, and the way persons respond to each other. The leader must also be aware of the group's communication with him or her, noting whether it is the same or different from the patterns among the followers.

Research has shown that group member satisfaction increases when the leader demonstrates confidence in group members' ability (Miles, 1975, p. 121). Confidence can be communicated to members by verbalizing the trust that the leader has in group members. For example, the leader can say, "I know that you will do a good job."

Group member satisfaction also increases as the frequency of consultations initiated by the leader increases (Miles, 1975, p. 120). That is, group members like to be asked about their opinions and approaches to situations in which they are expected to participate. The more the leader is able to communicate with the group, the more satisfied the members will be.

Assertiveness

A second important attribute for the effective leader is assertiveness. Assertiveness can be viewed on a continuum as shown in Figure 2-1. A leader's behavior may be classified as nonassertive, assertive, or aggressive. Of course no one behaves the same way all the time, so one can move along the continuum in either direction. The goal, however, is assertiveness.

Assertiveness includes expressing one's feelings, needs, and ideas, and standing up for one's rights, while considering the rights of others (Bloom, Coburn, & Pearlman, 1975, p. 8). Assertive persons establish close interpersonal relationships; protect them-

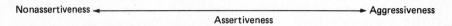

Figure 2-1 Assertiveness continuum.

selves from being used by others; make their own life decisions and choices; identify and meet many of their interpersonal needs; and express positive and negative feelings, both verbally and nonverbally (Cotler & Guerra, 1976, p. 3). Assertive persons generally feel good about themselves and others.

There are five ways for the leader to act assertively (Lange & Jakubowski, 1976, pp. 14-18). The first type of assertive behavior is using *basic assertion*, which is a simple statement of one's feelings, needs, or ideas. For this, no special communication skills are necessary. Basic assertion could be a simple "yes" or "no." In response to a request from a group member, the leader could say, "I will consider your request and let you know tomorrow."

Empathic assertion is the second type of assertive behavior. When using empathic assertion, the leader first gives recognition to the other person's feelings or situation and then makes a statement about his or her own position. A leader might say to the group, when they have not quite completed a task, but their work time is over, "I know you would really like to finish this today, but we cannot afford to give you overtime pay, so you will have to stop. We can finish it tomorrow."

A third type of assertive behavior is *escalating assertion.* Escalation is used when the other person fails to respond. It involves making successive assertive statements that gradually become more and more firm. The sentences may also become shorter and more blunt. In the following example, the leader uses a basic assertion, an empathic assertion, and then two firmer basic assertions.

> *Group member:* Hey, boss, it's Friday. Let's all go to Happy Hour.
> *Leader:* Thanks for asking, but I'd rather not.
> *Group member:* Oh, come on. Everyone is going.
> *Leader:* I know you would like everyone to be there, but I can't go.
> *Group member:* Just for a little while?
> *Leader:* No. Now please go.

When using escalating assertion, it must be remembered that an end point must come. Power struggles are apt to lead to aggressiveness. In the example above, the leader finally said, "Please go," to indicate a final response. If the leader thought that the member had some other unidentified need which had caused this continuing request, the leader might have decided to ask the member if there was some other issue the member wanted to discuss.

The fourth type of assertiveness is *confrontive assertion.* When a person's words contradict his or her actions, confrontive assertion may be used. The leader describes objectively what the other person agreed to do, what actually was done, and then what the leader wants. For example:

You told me that you would have the report in by noon on Thursday. It is now Friday morning, and I still don't have the report. I expect you to have it in my office by noon today.

I-language assertion is the fifth type of assertive behavior. The leader makes a four-part statement that includes: *when you do . . ., the effects on me are . . ., I feel . . .,* and *I would prefer. . . .* The purpose of this type of assertion is for the person to state his or her own feelings and expectations. It is most often used when the leader feels hurt or irritated. If a member of the group consistently comes late to meetings, the leader might appropriately say:

When you come late to the meetings, it disturbs my thinking and participation in the group. It makes me feel very frustrated and angry. I would prefer that you either come on time, or not come at all.

It is not always necessary or appropriate to use the "I feel" and "I would prefer" parts of the assertion. When they are not used, this is similar to a basic assertion, which may lead to the other person identifying a solution to the problem, or to both persons solving problems together. In the above example, the leader might have said, "When you consistently come late to meetings, I become very angry with you." The leader's feelings have been stated, but the statement has been left open for the follower to respond.

Nonassertiveness can be described as denying one's own feelings, needs, and ideas, ignoring one's own rights, or permitting others to infringe on one's rights (Bloom et al., 1975, p. 8). Nonassertive persons tend to put themselves down and let others make choices and decisions for them (Phelps & Austin, 1975, p. 11). People who are nonassertive usually behave this way to avoid conflict; however, they usually end up being angry—with others and with themselves.

Aggressiveness can be described as expressing one's feelings, needs and ideas at the expense of another person, standing up for one's own rights, but ignoring the rights of others, and trying to dominate and humiliate others (Bloom et al., 1975, p. 8). Aggressive persons just want to achieve their goals, but because of their methods, they often end up feeling bitter, guilty, and lonely.

Accountability

The third attribute for the effective leader is accountability. Leaders are accountable to themselves, their group, their profession, and their superiors. Accountability is answering to someone for the positive or negative outcomes of one's actions.

To be accountable to oneself, one must be able to objectively view what one is doing with one's work and one's life. In effect, a leader will believe that he or she is OK, but will be able to make alterations if deemed necessary. A person must feel satisfied with what he or she is doing, and feel good about it to be an effective leader.

To be accountable to the group, the leader must be able to tell members what has been done on their behalf. Accountability includes negative as well as positive elements. Therefore, a leader must also tell the group what he or she has failed to do. Making excuses is not accountability: the leader just presents facts. For example, a nurse is accountable to her patient when she tells the patient that she asked the doctor to order a medication that the patient had requested. She also is accountable to the patient when she tells the patient that she gave him or her the wrong medication.

Accountability to one's profession includes a willingness to judge one's professional peers and a conscientious development of the ability to judge (Passos, 1973, p. 18). As discussed in Chapter 1, a profession has standards and a code of ethics to which the members must adhere. The only way that standards can be developed, revised, and applied is through the judgment of the members of the profession. Judging professional peers, and being judged by them, is truly being accountable to the profession. An effective leader will be actively involved in peer evaluation.

Rarely do people function without some kind of superior or supervisor. Even the "top" boss of a company has a board of directors to whom he or she must respond. Consequently, a leader must be accountable to his or her superior, and answer for the work the leader and the group have or have not done. For example, a nursing team leader answers to the head nurse, who, in turn, answers to the nursing supervisor.

Advocacy

Finally, an effective leader is always an advocate for his or her group. An advocate supports, defends, and maintains the cause of someone or something. Advocacy has been called that part of a person's nature known as "selfish benevolence" (Kerschner, 1976, p. i). The leader-advocate works to change the power structure, so that the situation of his or her group or client, which may be socially, politically, economically, or otherwise deprived, is improved. In other words, an advocate assists a special interest group to achieve and use power effectively to produce certain desired societal changes (Berger, 1976, p. 2).

Advocacy has become an essential part of nursing leadership (Fay, 1978, p. 252). In nursing, the leader's group is often one or more patients. Whether the group is a single individual or a number of individuals, however, the leader-advocate functions in the same way. A staff nurse might discuss with the operating room supervisor the problem her patient had with the person who did the surgical shave. Or, a school nurse might recognize that teenage pregnancy is a problem in a particular community and work to establish a Planned Parenthood organization in the community. Both nurses have taken up the cause of assisting clients to meet their needs.

The *patient rights advocate* is a relatively new role that has developed within the health care system. The primary goal of this type of leader is to help patients understand their rights as patients and to see that they are afforded those rights (Annas, 1974, p. 21). While there has been some controversy regarding who should be the patient rights advocate, it is clear that the nurse-leader must assume the role.[1]

---

[1] The American Hospital Association has provided a bill of rights for patients in hospitals, which outlines what patients should expect regarding their care. Many hospitals have now made the American Hospital Association's bill of rights specific to their institutions. The patient rights advocate assists patients to obtain these rights. The nurse-leader should be familiar with the bill of rights used by her institution; if one does not exist, the nurse-leader should work for the development of such a document.

THE GROUP

The leader must have a relationship with a group; however, several more terms must be defined before proceeding with a discussion of the group. A group can be defined as a number of individuals working together to achieve a common goal. This type of group is a work group, i.e., the members are *working* together. A work group may consist of as few as two members—the leader and a follower (e.g., nurse and a client)—or it may consist of many members (e.g., the head nurse and the staff).

Group process refers to the changes that occur within the group as the members work together to achieve their goal, including how problems are identified, how goals are set, and how work is accomplished and evaluated. *Group dynamics* refers to the interacting forces and communication patterns among the members of a group; it includes such things as who talks with whom and how supportive members are to one another.

Group Development

When analyzing a group, the first thing to study is the growth of the group—its process and dynamics. Groups may be formed in many ways. When a nurse establishes a contract with a patient, a new group is formed; when a new nurse begins work on a particular unit, a new group is formed; when any nurse leaves a particular unit, a new group is formed. It can be seen that groups are begun and terminated every day.

The size of a group has an important effect on its development. A small group will form, achieve its task, and terminate much more quickly and informally than a large group. The process is speedier and the dynamics far less complex in a small group.

Much has been written about the phases of group development, and various labels have been given to the phases. Since a group is a series of interpersonal relationships, a convenient approach is to use the concept of growth—from dependent, to independent, to interdependent—an approach that is used to explain other interpersonal relationships.

The first phase of group development is the phase of *dependence*. Dependence refers to a need for support. During the dependent phase, members are becoming acquainted with each other. They are usually insecure and anxious, and feel the need for support. They also tend to be very ego-centered; they function alone and for their own benefit. Communication is being established, but members still think of themselves first. An observer of a group in this phase would hear a great deal of I-language, e.g., "I am," or "I think."

As the tension level in the group changes, the second phase, the phase of *independence*, begins. Members start to view the group as a group. However, they are still more conscious of their own place within the group than they are of the development of the group as a whole.

During this phase, the members become concerned with the organization of the group, and roles are established. If a leader is not present, one will usually be appointed, as well as a secretary and any other positions that are deemed necessary for the task. Very often members will volunteer for the positions available—an indication of their concern for being part of the group.

Limits will usually be placed, either implicitly or explicitly, on the degree of power these appointed persons will be given. Other rules of order for the group will also be established.

The third phase of group development is the phase of *interdependence*. Interdependence occurs when each member views the goals and purpose of the group as more important than individual preferences. In other words, the individuals have become a group. An observer would hear a great deal of group interaction such as, "We could . . .," "Let's . . .," or "How about . . . ," and the dynamics become very complex.

By this time the members have developed a sense of basic trust in one another. Since the members can relate personally to one another and experience trust, the group becomes a cohesive unit. Members can share their satisfactions and frustrations with the group, and have confidence in the group. A state of equilibrium has been reached.

The group process is directed toward problem solving, and group responsibilities are shared. Members feel a sense of responsibility to and for the group. Since they know that the group, like a chain, is only as strong as its weakest member, all members work hard for the group. High morale tends to be directly correlated with high production.

The time that it takes for the phases of group development is quite variable. The first phase is usually brief because it is so uncomfortable. The second phase may take longer as the distribution of power occurs. The third phase lasts the longest because it is the working phase, the time in which most of the work is done.

As mentioned before, the size of the group greatly affects the time it takes for group development. Obviously a group of two members will move rapidly through the phases, whereas a group of six or ten will take progressively more time.

Other factors also affect the time needed for group development. The importance and relevance of the task to the members has a great effect. If all members are willing and able to achieve the task, the process will be facilitated. If some members are neither willing nor able, the process will be slowed, since these members must be assisted to overcome their limitations.

The environment or physical location of the group affects the group's development. The environment should be comfortable and free from distractions. When a team conference is held on the nursing unit, nurses will find themselves running to answer patient lights, assist visitors, or perform other tasks. Consequently, group development will be hindered by the coming and going of individual members. If the team can meet in a private conference room, away from the activity of the unit (and the team has arranged for other nurses to cover for them during their absence) group development will be facilitated because all members will be present and participating.

The time allotted or available to the group will also affect the time it will take for group development. Frequent, even brief amounts of time are more beneficial than infrequent, long periods. A committee that meets once a month may spend most of its time in the dependence and independence phases because the members must become reacquainted each time the group meets. In contrast, nursing staff who work together nearly every day can move rapidly through the first two phases and focus on solving problems together.

One other factor that affects the time needed for group development is the previous experience in groups that each of the members has. Members who have had a good deal of experience in other groups can facilitate the developmental process for themselves and for the rest of the group. Members who have little or no prior group experience may hold back the process because they are unsure of what is happening.

In addition, members who have had good group experience in the past, regardless of the number, will be an asset to the group's development, since these members will have a sound base for understanding group development. Members who have had poor experiences may have difficulty adjusting to the new group, and may thus delay the developmental process.

Finally, a fourth phase of group development may be considered—the phase of *termination*. An effective group is able to dissolve or change itself when its purpose is achieved. For example, an ad hoc committee whose task is completed must dissolve itself. If the task has not been completed, the group may arrange to continue as an ad hoc committee or decide to become a standing committee of the organization.

Group members may feel sad, angry, guilty, or glad when the group ends. Social groups may develop from the group if some or all of the members choose to remain together. The length of the termination phase is proportional to the length of time the group has been together (Clark, 1977, p. 34).

Group Member Roles

Group members perform two types of roles, or functions, to facilitate group process, *task roles* and *maintenance roles*. Task roles have to do with the job at hand (i.e., meeting the goals and objectives) and getting it done as rapidly as possible. Maintenance roles are used to keep the group functioning happily and cohesively.

Task Roles

1 *Initiating* consists of beginning the discussion, or introducing a new part of the discussion. For example, "Today we are going to discuss. . . ."

2 *Giving information* includes presenting ideas, facts, or generalizations to the group and relating one's own experience to the problem under discussion. For example, "I cared for a woman who had that problem. For her it worked to. . . ."

3 *Asking for information* may be done to find answers to questions of which one is unsure. It may also be done to seek other solutions or to determine the ramifications of this solution. For example, "What would that involve?" Asking questions is one of the most important roles and often the most difficult. However, if there are no questions, there is literally no discussion.

4 *Giving reactions* to someone else's idea means sharing one's own beliefs or opinions about that idea. For example, "I believe X could happen if we do that."

5 *Clarifying* involves presenting information in different ways from the one in which it was presented. It may include elaborating the facts or presenting examples. Often, restating an idea will clarify it for oneself and for others. For example, "So you're saying: If we do X, Y will result."

6 *Synthesizing and summarizing* involve putting together what has been discussed and providing closure for an idea or topic. For example, "Now it seems that we have been saying. . . ." Summarizing keeps members of the group at the same point in the discussion.

7 *Orienting* means keeping the group focused on the topic of discussion or bringing them back if they do depart from the topic. For example, "That's very interesting, but we were talking about. . . ."

8 *Timekeeping* means helping the group to be aware of the passage of time, so that the discussion may be finished at the appointed time. For example, "We only have 10 minutes left." If specific time allotments have been set for various topics, timekeeping also includes watching the time for each topic.

Maintenance Roles

1 *Encouraging* is supporting another member and giving him or her credit for making a contribution. It includes being friendly and warm. For example, "Thank you. That is a good idea."

2 *Sponsoring* is assisting another member by asking that member to speak. For example, "We haven't heard from you yet, Pete. What do you think about X?" Sponsoring can be difficult, since others may feel it condescending, so the words used and the tone of voice are important. When a member is not actively participating, it is often better to ask a question to which the member knows the answer than to confront him or her with nonparticipation.

3 *Harmonizing* is an attempt to calm tense group feelings or to help others deal with their differences. It may include making light of something or pointing out the humor in the situation. For example, "Look what we're doing. We're getting really uptight about a minor point. We have better things to do." Or, "Let's table this until we have more time to reflect on it, and go on to something else."

4 *Compromising* is being willing to give in when you are involved in a disagreement. For example, "I hear what you are saying. Is there a middle ground where we could agree?"

5 *Standard setting* includes providing a goal for the group to achieve in terms of its functioning, and holding the group to that goal during evaluation of the group. For example, "During our meeting today let's be sure to really listen to each other."

Listening is not considered a specific role, but it is included in all the roles. An effective group member listens attentively at all times.

It must be remembered that these roles are not mutually exclusive, and any participation by a member may be a combination of roles. Further, *all* members of the group, not just the leader, are responsible for using the roles. In an effective, cohesive group, all members will feel free to perform all the roles at various times, and will also feel it their responsibility to see that all the roles are performed.

Members can also assume roles that work against the group process. Examples of nonfunctional roles include dominating (talking too much), withdrawing (not talking), competing between members, seeking sympathy for one's point of view, and manipulating others. It is important that these roles not be performed. If one member enacts one of these roles, another member should use a functional role to restore effective discussion.

Group Climate

Probably the most important factor in effective group functioning is the climate of the group. The climate is the feeling tone that is consistently present among the members.

Trust ←——→ Cohesiveness ←——→ Communication ←——→ Problem solving ————→ PRODUCTION

Figure 2-2   Group process is linear and results in productivity.

A climate of mutual trust and support leads to cohesiveness among members. Cohesiveness refers to the degree of commitment or loyalty that each member has for the group as a whole.

In a healthy group climate, every member is given respect and understanding by every other member. Members can share their strengths as well as their limitations, and still be accepted. Members feel free to contribute whatever they can, and know that the contribution will be viewed as their unique part in the process.

When the climate is good, productivity will be high. The purpose of a group is to achieve a goal, and when the goal has been met, the group has been productive. Achievement of the goal is therefore the expected output, or production.

Production is achieved through the processes of problem solving and decision making. (See Chapter 7 for a thorough discussion of decision making.) These processes occur only when the group dynamics are good, i.e., there is a high degree of interaction and communication. Communication is fostered by a climate of trust and a cohesive group. Therefore group process may be viewed as a linear process, as shown in Figure 2-2.

Group Problems

Regardless of how cohesive and productive a group is, some problems will always occur. It is important for the leader to be prepared to deal with problems, when they appear. Areas of difficulty are many and varied, and depend on the specific group, but certain problems are likely to be encountered in any group. These may be classified as follows:

1 *Interpersonal problems* are the most obvious and most common group problems. Poor communication techniques, use of nonfunctional roles, personality conflicts, and prejudice are examples.

2 *Addition or loss of members* changes the group and may therefore create feelings of tension. Dynamics are affected, as is the power structure. Members may miss an old member very much and, as a result, fail to accept a new member into the group.

3 *Intergroup problems* happen when the goals of two groups differ—mildly, or to a greater degree. When the groups are in conflict, problems may arise within each group. For example, nurses in a coronary care unit constitute one group, nurses on a postcoronary unit another. If the two groups do not carry out the same protocols for cardiac rehabilitation, conflicts will arise. Furthermore, the nurses may become upset with members of their own group because some will be doing things in one way and some in another.

4 *Intrapersonal problems* are those that occur within a person. Individual group members may cause problems for the group because of problems they bring with them from their homes, families, or elsewhere. For example, worry for a sick child at home or marital problems affect one's entire behavior (including behavior in the group), and not just the relationship directly involved. Another intrapersonal problem that may affect the group may occur when goals of one group conflict with goals of another group to which a member belongs. For example, a Roman Catholic nurse who works

on a gynecology unit where elective abortions are performed may feel conflict between her religious goals and her nursing unit goals.

These problems all relate to conflicts, and conflict management is an important strategy for a leader to use. It is dealt with specifically in Chapter 10.

Group Evaluation

Groups must be consistently evaluated to determine how well they are functioning. The leader and each member, individually and collectively, should be involved in evaluation. Criteria on which a group may be evaluated include the following:

1 The group has a clear understanding of its goals.
2 Group goals and needs are integrated with individual goals and needs.
3 All members use task and maintenance roles.
4 Members are loyal to the group.
5 The group sets and achieves realistic goals.
6 Effective problem solving and decision making occur.
7 A variety of resources are used by the group.
8 The potential of each individual is utilized to the fullest.
9 The group objectively evaluates itself.
10 The group is flexible and can function within the regulation of the larger group.
11 Responsibilities are shared among members.

Evaluation is an important process that provides feedback to group members and to the larger group they serve. Periodic evaluation during the group's development and work aids in accomplishing the original group goal. Evaluation will be further discussed in Chapter 11.

SUMMARY

Two important concepts in the study of leadership are the leader and the group. This discussion has emphasized four essential attributes of the effective leader—awareness, assertiveness, accountability, and advocacy. These attributes enable the leader to relate to and influence the group. Group process and group dynamics were discussed to show some of the complexities involved in working with a group. The interaction of the leader with the group makes goal setting and goal achievement possible.

REFERENCES

Annas, G. F. The patient rights advocate: Can nurses effectively fill the role? *Supervisor Nurse*, 1974, 5(7), 20–25.

Berger, M. An orienting perspective on advocacy. In P. A. Kerschner (Ed.), *Advocacy and age*. Los Angeles: Andrus Gerontology Center, 1976.

Bloom, L. Z., Coburn, K., & Pearlman, J. *The new assertive woman*. New York: Delacorte, 1975.

Clark, C. C. *The nurse as group leader.* New York: Springer, 1977.

Cotler, S. B., & Guerra, J. J. *Assertive training.* Champaign, Ill.: Research Press, 1976.

Fay, P. Sounding board in support of patient advocacy as a nursing role. *Nursing Outlook*, 1978, *26*, 252–253.

Goldstein, A. P., & Sorcher, M. *Changing supervisor behavior.* New York: Pergamon, 1974.

Hersey, P., & Blanchard, K. H. *Management of organizational behavior utilizing human resources.* Englewood Cliffs, N.J.: Prentice-Hall, 1977.

Hollander, E. P. Emergent leadership and social influence. In L. Petrullo & B. M. Bass (Eds.), *Leadership and interpersonal behavior.* New York: Holt, Rinehart, & Winston, 1961.

Hollander, E. P. *Leaders, groups, and influence.* New York: Oxford University Press, 1964.

Kerschner, P. A. (Ed.). *Advocacy and age.* Los Angeles: Andrus Gerontology Center, 1976.

Lange, A. J., & Jakubowski, P. *Responsible assertive behavior.* Champaign, Ill.: Research Press, 1976.

Miles, R. E. *Theories of management: Implications for organizational behavior and development.* New York: McGraw-Hill, 1975.

Passos, J. Y. Accountability: Myth or mandate? *Journal of Nursing Administration*, 1973, *3*(3), 17–22.

Phelps, S., & Austin, N. *The assertive woman.* Fredericksburg, Va.: Book Crafters, 1975.

ADDITIONAL READINGS

Benne, K. D., & Sheats, P. Functional roles of group members. *Journal of Social Issues*, 1948, *4*(2), 41–49.

Bion, W. R. *Experiences in groups.* New York: Basic Books, 1959.

Bradford, L. P. (Ed.). *Group development.* La Jolla, Calif.: University Associates, 1978.

Cartwright, D., & Zander, A. (Eds.). *Group dynamics.* New York: Harper & Row, 1968.

Cooper, S. S. Methods of teaching revisited: Informal discussion. *Journal of Continuing Education in Nursing*, 1978, *9*(5), 14–16.

Corona, D. F. Followership: The indispensable corollary to leadership. *Nursing Leadership*, 1979, *2*(2), 5–8.

Diekelmann, N. L., & Broadwell, M. M. How to get the job done . . . by someone else. *Nursing '77*, 1977, *7*(9), 110–116.

Diers, D. Lessons on leadership. *Image*, 1979, *11*, 67–71.

Garnett, J. What is leadership? *Nursing Mirror and Midwives Journal*, 1976, *143*(14), 40–41.

Gordon, T. *Group-centered leadership.* Chicago: Houghton Mifflin, 1955.

Gorman, A. H. *The leader in the group.* New York: Teacher's College, Columbia University, 1963.

Knowles, M., & Knowles, H. *Introduction to group dynamics.* New York: Association Press, 1972.

Larson, M. L., & Williams, R. A. How to become a better group leader? *Nursing '78*, 1978, *8*(8), 65–72.

Layden, M. Responsibility to self: First step to leadership. *Nursing Leadership*, 1979, *2*(3), 26–29.

Luft, J. *Group processes*. Palo Alto, Calif.: National Press Books, 1970.

McNally, J. M. Leadership–the needed component. *Nursing Leadership*, 1979, *2*(3), 6–12.

Munn, H. E., Jr. Measure your nursing supervisor leadership behaviors. *Hospital Topics*, 1976, *54*(6), 14–18.

Parker, T. "What's a nice person like you doing to people?" *Hospital Topics*, 1979, *57*(1), 32–37.

Patton, B. R., & Giffin, K. *Decision-making group interaction*. New York: Harper & Row, 1978.

Sampson, E. E., & Marthas, M. S. *Group process for the health professions*. New York: Wiley, 1977.

Schein, E. H. *Organizational psychology*. Englewood Cliffs, N.J.: Prentice-Hall, 1970.

Shaw, M. E. *Group dynamics: The psychology of small group behavior*. New York: McGraw-Hill, 1976.

Shores, L. Staff development for leadership. *Nursing Clinics of North America*, 1978, *13*, 103–109.

Tead, O. *The art of leadership*. New York: McGraw-Hill, 1935.

Uris, A. *Techniques of leadership*. New York: McGraw-Hill, 1953.

Zorn, J. M. Nursing leadership for the 70s and 80s. *Journal of Nursing Administration*, 1977, *7*(8), 33–35.

Chapter 3

The Organization

The concept of organization comes from business and management. Organization originally meant the process of *organizing* an *organization*. Organizing is one of the functions in the managerial theory of leadership, and is now considered an important leadership strategy, one which will be discussed in Chapter 6. Organization refers to the institution itself, the setting in which the leader (for our purposes, the nurse-leader) functions, and it is the focus of this chapter.

ORGANIZATIONAL THEORY

To understand the organization of a health care agency, e.g., a hospital, nursing home, or public health department, or of any other kind of institution, one must be familiar with organizational theory. It is generally accepted that there are three principal theories of organization—classical, humanistic, and modern.

Classical Doctrine

Classical doctrine is the oldest theory of organization. It emphasizes rigid, centralized control of workers to promote high production. An institution organized under classical theory tends to treat workers in a mechanical, yet objective way. The institution is very efficient, and effective in accomplishing its goals.

Frederick Taylor is considered the founder of classical theory and is known as "the father of scientific management." High production was his primary concern in developing the theory. Taylor believed that high production could be achieved by paying high wages. In his opinion, it was possible to pay high wages and still have an overall low labor cost (Taylor, 1911, p. 22). Obviously the labor cost had to be low for the institution to make a profit.

Scientific management, Taylor's approach, involves timing various work activities with a stopwatch. The purpose is to determine the exact time in which a worker should be able to accomplish a task. Workers should be given a large task, but one they are able to accomplish. For example, if a worker works 8 hours, he or she should be given a task that takes exactly 8 hours to complete. Workers are rewarded with high pay for successfully accomplishing the task, but disciplined if they fail to accomplish it (Taylor, 1911, pp. 63–64).

Further, in the classical approach, strict obedience to authority is expected. Workers must do the "hand work" exactly as they are told to do it by their superior. Only top-level managers may do "brain work," because this type of work is not directly related to increasing production. The workers' job is to keep production going.

Fayol identified fourteen principles of management and further developed Taylor's ideas (Fayol, 1949, pp. 19–41). The principles made it clear that production, efficiency, and profit were of prime importance, while individuals, or workers, were of little importance.

Division of work, the first principle, is the root of classical doctrine, from which everything else develops. Division of work, or specialization, happens as an organization grows and there is more work to do. If the work is divided so that each person has only one task to do, the cost of production will be lower.

Fayol's principles are as follows:[1]

1 *Division of work.* Work is broken down into specialized tasks.

2 *Authority.* Employers have the right to give orders and expect them to be obeyed.

3 *Discipline.* The employee is expected to be obedient to the institution.

4 *Unity of command.* An employee should receive orders from only one superior.

5 *Unity of direction.* There is only one person at the top of the institution, and he or she has only one plan for the institution.

6 *Subordination of individual interests to general interest.* Institutional goals and activities always come first.

7 *Remuneration of personnel.* Salary should be fair and, as far as possible, satisfactory to both employer and employee.

8 *Centralization.* All communication comes from, and goes to, the person at the top of the institution.

9 *Scalar chain.* There is a chain of superiors, ranging from the person at the top, down to the employee at the bottom of the institution.

10 *Order.* There is a place for everyone, and everyone must be in his place.

---

[1] Fayol's principles of management, with interpretations. Source: H. Fayol. *General and industrial management.* London: Pitman, 1949. Used by permission.

11 *Equity.* All persons in the institution will be treated alike.

12 *Stability of tenure for personnel.* A prosperous institution has a stable group of workers.

13 *Initiative.* Within the limits of respect for authority and discipline, any employee has the freedom to propose and execute a plan.

14 *Esprit de corps.* In union there is strength.

A worker who does only one task becomes highly skilled and efficient, and will be able to do the task faster and faster; therefore, production will increase. In addition, if he or she is replaced, it is cheaper and faster to train someone else to do one small task than to do a more complex combination of tasks.

As each worker becomes specialized and the organization grows, the scalar chain develops. To retain control, the top manager establishes discipline and order. Likewise, the other principles follow from division of work. Concern for workers must be present to a degree, or the organization will fall apart. Consequently, equity and esprit de corps are included in the principles—but at the bottom of the list where they can easily be forgotten or omitted.

Humanistic School

It was the demonstrated lack of concern for workers which led to the formulation of a new theory of organization in the 1930s. The humanistic theory, also called behavioral or neoclassical theory, identifies two major functions of organizations. One is *maintaining the external balance*, i.e., the economics (the focus of classical theory). The other is *maintaining the internal balance*, i.e., the social organization of the workers, through which they satisfy their own desires and needs by working together (Roethlisberger & Dickson, 1939, p. 552). These two functions have equal importance in humanistic theory.

Humanists recognize that workers have a collectivity of their own simply because they are in contact with and interact with each other. This collectivity is called the informal organization, in contrast to the formal organization, or the workers as a unit within the total organization (Roethlisberger & Dickson, 1939, p. 511). Though it has no formal structure, the informal organization has three specific functions: (1) communication among workers, (2) maintenance of cohesiveness among workers through a willingness to serve and to accept authority, and (3) maintenance of feelings of personal integrity, self-respect, and independent choice (Barnard, 1938, p. 122).

Humanistic theory also recognizes that an individual's goals may differ from the overall organizational goals. An institution organized according to humanistic theory therefore allows and encourages participation of workers in planning and decision making. The institution tries to promote general job satisfaction for workers because, according to this theory, concern for workers' needs, as well as for profit and production, will lead to improved production and economic effectiveness.

Modern Organizational Theory

Modern organizational theory began in the late 1950s and early 1960s, as researchers recognized that, in the humanistic as well as in the classical approach, something was missing. Researchers have taken several different approaches to modern organizational theory and consequently the theory is still evolving and is not that well integrated. Modern organizational theory is also called *systems theory, management science, matrix theory*, or *organic theory*. Modern organizational theory comes from sociology, psychology, economics, and mathematics. Because of the popularity of systems theory, it appears that the subtheories will eventually merge into a systems framework (Woodward, 1965).

The basic assumption of modern organizational theory in a systems framework is that an organization is an open system, consisting of input, throughput, output, and feedback. The task of management is to trace the pattern of energy exchange, i.e., the activities of workers, as it results in output, and then to ascertain how the output is translated back into energy to reactivate the system (Katz & Kahn, 1966, p. 18). The parts of the system may be identified as the individual, the formal organization, the status and role arrangements in the organization, and the setting of the organization (Scott & Mitchell, 1972, p. 57).

Communication is viewed as an extremely important process in modern organizational theory, since it facilitates the interdependence of all parts of the system. It is the "mechanism of coordination" (Rogers & Agarwala-Rogers, 1976, p. 57). An institution that utilizes modern organizational theory emphasizes horizontal as well as vertical communication because all parts of the institution are parts of the system and are therefore essential to each other.

Because of the way it is evolving, modern organizational theory has a synthesizing and integrating nature. Furthermore, it is highly analytical and has the advantage of being based on empirical research (Scott & Mitchell, 1972, p. 55).

Relationships among Theories

The three types of organizational theories are closely related. Humanistic theory builds on classical, and modern organizational theory builds on both classical and humanistic. Classical theory considers only the formal organization; humanistic theory considers the individual as well as the formal and informal organizations; and modern organizational theory considers all those, plus status, role arrangements, and setting. Institutions may use one theory exclusively, or may use parts of theories as a basis for their operations.

USE OF ORGANIZATIONAL THEORIES BY HEALTH CARE FACILITIES

It is important for the nurse-leader to know the theory of organization used by the health care facility in which she functions. The treatment of employees is determined by the theory and, based on that determination, the nurse-leader may decide whether or not she wishes to work in that facility.

Most hospitals and public health agencies are still organized primarily according to the classical approach, that is, high production (patient care) at a low labor cost is the major consideration. Most health care facilities do not exist to make a profit, but financial stability is still of great concern.

Many hospitals have done time and motion studies (i.e., studies to assess the time required and used to do various activities) to determine nurse-patient care ratios. When a hospital administrator determines, through such studies, that a 1 to 5 nurse-patient ratio is necessary, he or she is using the principles of scientific management.

Most hospitals still have a centralized organizational structure. All authority and communication comes from, and goes to, the top level. What this often means for employees is frustration, since they have little or no voice in planning and decision making.

Some health care facilities try to use the humanistic approach. Though still centralized, such institutions may try to decrease the number of levels in the institution. For example, if a hospital's hierarchy consisted of director, supervisor, head nurse, assistant head nurse, and staff nurse, the associate director and the assistant head nurse might be eliminated in an attempt to humanize the institution. However, it is likely that, even with the elimination of two levels, the organization will still be quite centralized with regard to authority and communication.

Another possibility is that some departments in an institution *are* humanistic, while others, including the central hospital administration, remain classical (Lippitt, 1973, p. 57). When the nurse-leader is interviewed by the director of nursing for a position in such a hospital, she may be told that the hospital has a humanistic, or employee-oriented organization. However, when the nurse-leader talks with staff nurses who function in the hospital, she may get quite a different viewpoint.

Health care facilities that want to be humanistic recognize the informal organization, or "grapevine." To minimize the effects of the grapevine, administrators may ask employees for opinions regarding plans and changes. However, communication is still only allowed with one's immediate supervisor. For example, the staff nurse-employee gives her suggestions to her supervisor, and so on up the line.

Few health care facilities have attempted to organize according to modern organizational theory, possibly because administrators are comfortable with the classical hierarchy. It appears, however, that hospitals and hospital administrators in the future will have to use a modern or systems framework for organization. Development of human resources through mutual confidence rather than through obedience to authority is a key responsibility for modern hospitals (Lippitt, 1973, p. 59). A systems or matrix form of organization is the only way to achieve this goal. Hospital employees must have freedom of access to information, and greater communication is needed between and among all parts of the organization (Lippitt, 1973, p. 60).

The nurse-leader, then, considers the type of organization in which she will work. She determines how she, as an individual, will be treated: like a machine (classical), as a member of the informal organization (humanistic), or as one part of a complete system (modern). She identifies the communication patterns and the amount of input she will have in decisions. Based on her analysis, the nurse-leader may decide to join, or not to join, any particular institution.

ORGANIZATIONAL STRUCTURE

Organizational structure is a framework for the working relationships among members of an organization (Jucius, Deitzer, & Schlender, 1973, p. 216). It is a systematic arrangement of the work of an organization intended to ensure that the sum total of the activity of the organization accomplishes the objective of the organization (Sexton, 1970, p. 23). An organizational chart, also called an *organigram*, is a visual representation, or blueprint, of the organizational structure. It shows the positions within an institution, and their relationships to one another. Figures 3-1 to 3-8 are all examples of organizational charts. Often an organizational chart represents only part of an organization, as shown in Figure 3-1.

Although there is always a physical and psychological separation between members of an organization, all members must realize the importance of the total organization. Unless one sees the organization as a whole and realizes one's own small part in it, one cannot criticize it.

Some departments in health care facilities, nursing in particular, feel that only *their* work is important, or that their work is the most important. But *all* work is important, and must be accomplished satisfactorily for the objective to be reached and for the organization as a whole to be successful. For example, in a public health department, the main objective—the health of the community—cannot be achieved without the nursing, medical, environmental health, and laboratory divisions. In a hospital, care of patients cannot be accomplished without nursing, pharmacy, dietary, maintenance and other departments. The nurse-leader can help others to understand that, in order for all the objectives of the total institution to be achieved, their work must be synchronized with the work of those doing complementary jobs (Sexton, 1970, p. 12).

Scalar Chain and Functional Process

Several concepts are important to organizational structure. First, the scalar chain and the functional process—the vertical and horizontal growth of an organization—must be considered. The scalar chain is vertical growth, the functional process horizontal growth. The scalar chain consists of a number of levels or steps in the structure, i.e., the hierarchy. It refers to the grading of duties according to the degree of authority and responsibility given. The functional process is a division into different kinds of duties on the same level (Davis, 1977, p. 197).

In Figure 3-1, positions B, D, and H are divided by the scalar chain. The director of nursing, the assistant director of medical, and the head nurse of the emergency room have different positions, which are on different levels and which have very different responsibilities. The figure shows that positions E and F are divided by the functional process. The assistant director of surgical (E) and the assistant director of obstetrics and pediatrics (F) are on the same level and have similar authority and similar job descriptions, but they have different duties.

Line and Staff

The second important concept is that of line and staff. The line organization is the hierarchy of personnel that extends from the executive at the top of the organization to the workers at the bottom (Davis, 1951, p. 325). The "line" is often considered the backbone of an organization, since line workers are responsible for performing or supervising the direct, primary functions, i.e., creation, finance, and distribution of a good or service of the organization (Scott & Mitchell, 1972, p. 40).

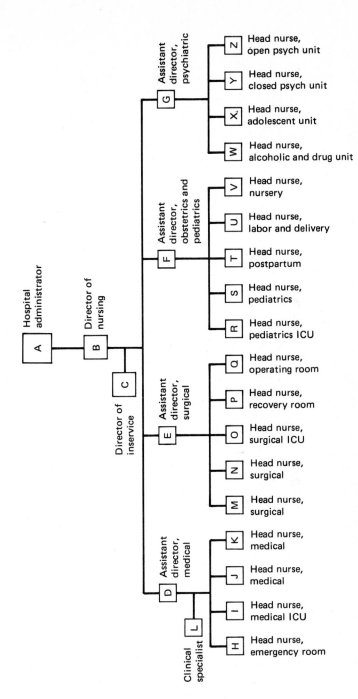

Figure 3-1 Nursing department organizational chart.

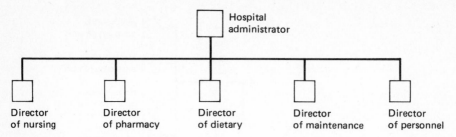

Figure 3-2 Hospital organizational chart.

The staff organization is developed to assist the line organization in some phase of its functioning (Davis, 1951, p. 370). Staff workers are expected to advise and serve the line workers. Their work should facilitate the work of line workers, and line workers should consult with staff workers. Staff workers may have to "sell" their ideas, however, because they have no final rights of decision and command (Davis, 1951, p. 435).

In Figure 3-1, A, B, G, and Z are all line workers; C and L are the only staff workers. Usually, on an organizational chart, line positions are connected by vertical lines, and staff positions are connected either by horizontal, or by dotted or broken lines.

Many conflicts and much confusion exist regarding line and staff. Another way of looking at the differences between line and staff is in terms of relationships instead of functions. Line positions exist along a direct line of authority—a superior-subordinate relationship—while the staff relationship is advisory only.

Line and staff also refer to persons, not departments. Although an organizational chart exists for the total institution, the head of a department may be the only person identified on the chart, as shown in Figure 3-2. Consequently, a departmental organizational chart often exists to make the relationships explicit within the department.

This approach can be taken a step further; only the head nurse may be identified on the chart, as illustrated in Figure 3-1. A nursing unit organizational chart may then be prepared to show the relationships in that specific unit of the nursing department (see Figures 3-6 to 3-8).

In nursing there is a specific problem related to line and staff. Most first-level nurses, i.e., the workers at the bottom of the organization, are called *staff* nurses. They are, however, in a *line* position because they carry out the main work of the organization.

Span of Control

Another concept related to organizational structure is span of control, which refers to the number of persons a manager can effectively supervise. Classical theory kept the span short, i.e., the manager was given a small number of workers to supervise, because of the belief in rigid control over workers. A short span leads to what is called a tall, centralized, organizational structure, and a wide span leads to a flat, decentralized structure.

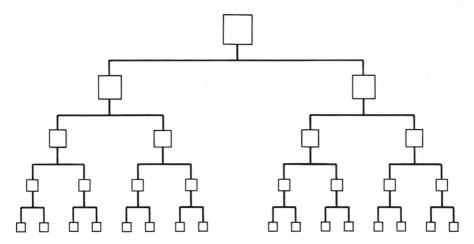

Figure 3-3 A centralized (tall) organization.

Figures 3-3 and 3-4 are both examples of thirty-one-person organizations. In Figure 3-3, the span of control is two, because each person supervises only two other workers, and there are five levels—a tall organization. In Figure 3-4, the span is five, and there are only three levels—a flatter and more decentralized organization.

There are advantages and disadvantages to both centralized and decentralized organizations. The centralized, or tall, organization, is advantageous for the manager, because it allows close coordination and control of workers. A disadvantage of a tall structure is that, because of the number of levels, communication from the bottom to the top of the organization is often difficult, and messages do not always get to the top. Another consequence is that workers tend to be very "boss-oriented" because of the close contact with their supervisor.

Being boss-oriented may have good or bad effects. High production is fostered when the boss is a good role model. However, little individual or original thinking occurs among boss-oriented workers.

The decentralized, or flat, organizational structure is advantageous for the worker. Because of the increased number of workers the supervisor must oversee, each worker is given more authority with less supervision. Communication chains are also shorter,

Figure 3-4 A decentralized (flat) organization.

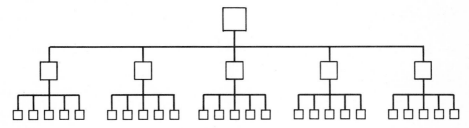

and workers are usually happier than those in a tall organization. The disadvantage of a flat organization is that the supervisor must oversee a larger number of workers; consequently, he or she cannot spend as much time in direct contact with each worker.

Responsibility, Authority, Delegation, and Accountability

Organizational structure cannot be studied without considering the concepts of responsibility, authority, delegation, and accountability. These four concepts are inseparable. Responsibility, which comes first, is the obligation to do, to the best of one's ability, the task that has been assigned, or delegated. In any organization, responsibility begins with the overall objective of the organization. For example, in a hospital, the overall objective may be service or patient care. In that case, patient care is the responsibility, which is delegated down the line to the various workers.

Authority—the right of decision and command—must be considered next. An individual who has authority has the right to make decisions about his or her own responsibilities, and the right to carry out those responsibilities or to require someone else to do so. Authority and power are different, though related; authority is a right, and power is the moral or physical force that maintains the right (Davis, 1951, p. 287).

Responsibility and authority are delegated down the scalar chain. Delegation is the process of assigning duties or responsibilities, along with corresponding authority, to another person.[2] Authority *must* be delegated with the responsibility, or in fact, one has not delegated.

Accountability is answering to someone for what has been done. It is related to responsibility because it involves reporting whether one has, or has not, carried out the responsibility assigned. Accountability cannot be delegated, since only the individual can choose to be, or not to be, accountable.

For example, a public health nurse (PHN) has the responsibility for the care of a caseload of patients. She herself need not see each patient more than once a month, so she assigns, or delegates, the care of a particular patient to a home health aide (HHA). The PHN also delegates to the HHA the necessary authority to care for the patient.

The HHA, in turn, carries out the assigned duties (her responsibility), and then reports back (accounts) to the PHN what she did. If the HHA arrived at the patient's home and found the patient lying on the floor because he or she had fallen, the HHA would call the PHN. She did not have authority to manage an emergency situation. The PHN could then delegate appropriate authority for any further responsibility that she might assign to the HHA.

NURSING DELIVERY SYSTEMS

Nursing delivery systems are types of organizations at the unit level. The nurse-leader must consider all the components of organization, regardless of the delivery system in which she functions.

---

[2] A more comprehensive discussion about delegation can be found in Chapter 6.

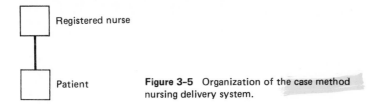

Figure 3-5 Organization of the case method nursing delivery system.

Case Method

Historically, in the United States, the case method was the first nursing delivery system. In the case method, a nurse works with only one patient, and meets all that patient's needs. Originally, the nurse actually lived with the patient in his or her home or hospital room, providing 24-hour care. The case method has developed, over the years, into the specialty of private duty nursing.

Today, private duty nursing is a disappearing specialty, but the private duty nurses remaining, many of whom are in their late fifties and sixties, still talk about their "cases." The case method, or modifications of it, is used today in emergency rooms and by nursing students, as well as by the remaining private duty nurses.

The organization of the case method is very simple, as Figure 3-5 shows. A one-to-one situation gives the nurse direct control of the patient and allows her to coordinate the patient's care. This is similar to a classical organization.

Advantages of the case method are that patients have very close relationships with their nurses, and their needs are likely to be met quickly. A great disadvantage is the cost; one registered nurse per patient makes costs very high. A major disadvantage in the past was the lack of personal and social life for the nurse, who might have only 2 hours off in 24 hours. This does not happen today, since a patient may have as many as three private duty nurses—one for each 8-hour shift.

Functional Method

During the Depression, nursing changed from a situation in which the majority of workers were private practitioners (private duty nurses in the case method) to one in which the workers were employees (Bullough & Bullough, 1969, p. 193). At the time, most hospitals had schools of nursing and utilized students as their employees. But, as nursing education developed to a point where student experiences were learning experiences, students could no longer be expected to function as employees and manage the hospital.

The advances in technology and medicine made patient care more complex, and hospitals recognized the need for graduate nurses. The number of patients requiring hospitalization also increased because medicine had become more scientific and could offer treatment within a hospital that often could not be offered at home.

Many former private duty nurses sought employment in hospitals because they needed to work. But, although the number of nurses employed by hospitals increased, the majority of nurses disliked hospital nursing. The reason for this was the amount of

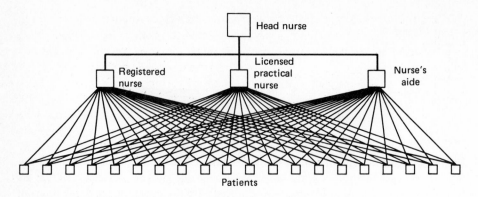

Figure 3-6 Organization of the functional nursing delivery system.

control the hospital exerted on the personal and professional lives of its employees (Bullough & Bullough, 1969, p. 194).

Hospitals were organized according to the classical theory, with each worker performing a specific task. Although graduate nurses were trained to handle every aspect of patient care, it was economically advantageous to assign tasks requiring little skill or education to personnel hired to assist the graduate nurses. These assistants, or nurse's aides, performed many tasks and cost the hospital less money than graduate nurses.

The shortage of graduate or registered nurses became critical during World War II, when many nurses left the hospitals and went to care for the soldiers. Consequently, hospitals were left with few nurses, who were assisted by nurse's aides and volunteers. It then became clear that nurses performed many different tasks or functions. Because of the limited number of registered nurses, the functional method for delivery of nursing service was further developed.

In the functional method, nursing is divided into its tasks, and different people do different tasks, e.g., nurse's aides make all the beds, licensed practical nurses give all the treatments, and registered nurses give all the medications. A head nurse is the supervisor over all, and it is to her that everyone else reports. The organizational chart for the functional method looks like Figure 3-6.

The functional method is similar to the classical organization in that all the responsibility and authority is delegated from the top. Responsibilities are arranged according to the functional process.

Advantages of the functional method include its efficiency, which is true of any classical organization. The method makes it possible to complete a great many tasks in a reasonable amount of time. Another possible advantage is that staff (registered nurses, licensed practical nurses, and nurse's aides) do only what they are capable of doing, or educated to do, but in practice this depends on the actual staff available.

The major disadvantage is that care of *persons* becomes fragmented. Patients do not know who their nurse is; in fact they have no nurse, they have three or four nurses, who may all say, "Someone else will do it."

Another disadvantage is that, because all nursing staff must communicate with the head nurse, the head nurse has little time to communicate with patients. Disadvantages for registered nurses include the fact that, although they are doing some of the tasks that they are prepared to do, i.e., giving medications and treatments, they are not doing others, i.e., personal care and communication. They do not have time for the latter, and that frustrates some and leads to reality shock in others.

The functional system is still used in some organizations. It is beneficial when staffing is poor, and thus tends to be used on weekends and on night shifts in large hospitals. It is also used in many small hospitals and nursing homes.

Many critical care units use a combination of the case and functional methods. One nurse cares for one or two patients; they are usually in the same room, and the nurse remains in the room with the patient(s) at all times. Many tasks, such as passing all medications or weighing patients, are assigned to another nurse who is not responsible for the care of any particular clients.

Team Nursing

Team nursing, which is used in many health care agencies today, was designed by Lambertson (1953) as a method of eliminating the fragmentation which resulted from the functional method. The idea underlying team nursing is that of working together democratically as a group.

A registered nurse team leader is assigned to the care of a group of patients. A group of staff members, e.g., one registered nurse, one licensed practical nurse, and one nurse's aide, are also assigned to the team leader. With a full knowledge of the needs, abilities, goals, and feelings of both the patients and the staff members, the team leader delegates the care of each patient to one particular staff member. Ideally that staff member will be stimulated to use her potential, since she will be the staff member most qualified to meet the needs of that particular patient. For example, a nurse's aide with 8 years of experience who likes to care for older male patients might be assigned to an 80-year-old, lucid, ambulatory male who, on a particular day, was being transferred back to the nursing home from which he entered the hospital.

The team leader is responsible for supervising and coordinating all the care given by her team members. She assists as necessary and meets any needs which she or another staff member identifies, but which the other staff member is unprepared to meet. The team leader is the only person who reports to the head nurse.

Team conferences are an important part of team nursing. The purpose of team conferences is to utilize the knowledge and skills of each team member in planning care for specific patients. Each team member's input is considered important.

The organization of team nursing appears in Figure 3-7. It can be considered a centralized organization with a tall structure. There is a narrow span of control, so that close supervision is assured. In any given hospital, on a particular nursing unit, two or more teams may be functioning, depending upon the number of patients and staff.

The major advantage of team nursing is that each team member's capabilities are utilized to the fullest, so that job satisfaction should be high. When nurses feel good about their jobs, patients will be given better care.

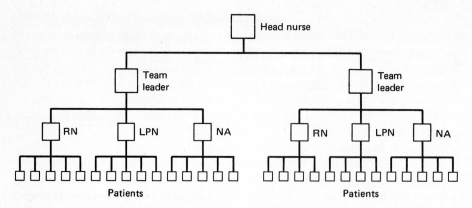

Figure 3-7 Organization of the team nursing delivery system.

In addition, the head nurse must meet only with team leaders, leaving her time to communicate with patients and do the overall supervision of the unit. Patients have one known nurse assigned to them, but they also see a registered nurse team leader, and perhaps the head nurse as well.

One disadvantage of team nursing is that, if a nurse who does not believe in team work, and who does not delegate, is assigned to be a team leader, the whole system may fall apart. Another disadvantage is that if the job of team leader is rotated among all registered nurses, a registered nurse may be a team leader one day and a team member the next. This can be confusing and frustrating. In addition, because nurses have days off, team composition varies from day to day, and this variance can be a disadvantage.

Primary Nursing

The newest approach to the delivery of nursing services was developed by Manthey (1970). Primary nursing was designed as a return to the concept of "my patient-my nurse." In this system, each registered nurse is assigned to the care of a group of patients for which she plans complete 24-hour care and writes the nursing care plan.

The primary nurse cares for her patients every time she works, for as long as the patients stay on her unit (ideally from admission through discharge). When she is not there, an associate nurse is assigned to the care of her patients, and will follow the primary nurse's care plans.[3]

The head nurse's role is very important, for she must assign new patients to the primary nurses, based on her assessment of the patient's needs and her knowledge of the primary nurse's present patients and her capabilities, preferences, needs, and goals. The head nurse communicates with primary nurses when they seek advice, but generally she delegates complete authority to them for the care of their patients.

---

[3] The primary nurse may choose *not* to care for one of her patients for a day if she has reason to believe that this would be beneficial. An associate nurse would then care for that patient for that day.

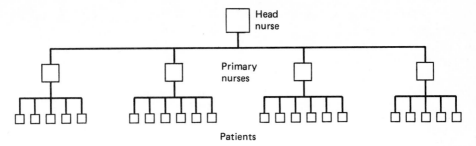

Figure 3-8 Organization of the primary nursing delivery system.

Licensed practical nurses function as associate nurses, and are supervised by the head nurse. When nursing assistants are used in a primary nursing system, they are generally assigned to assist primary and associate nurses by doing specific tasks for each nurse they assist.

The organization of primary nursing is shown in Figure 3-8. It is a more decentralized organizational structure than the other nursing delivery systems, and each primary nurse has greater responsibility and authority.

The main advantage of primary nursing is that it provides satisfaction for both patients and nurses. Patients know their nurses and are more apt to have their needs met. Nurses know their patients and feel a sense of accomplishment for giving complete care.

Moreover, primary nursing can be viewed as a nursing delivery system that is more professionalized than the other systems. Since the primary nurse is planning and providing complete care, she communicates with all other health team members involved in the client's care, and she provides for continuity of care. Other health team members tend to view the primary nurse as more knowledgeable and more responsible for the client.

Primary nurses *do* tend to be more knowledgeable about their clients, as well as more accountable; therefore, one would expect them to provide better quality of care. In addition, primary nurses are more satisfied because they continue their learning as they provide in-depth care to clients. Primary nursing is more like the care that nursing students give and, because of this similarity, many new graduate nurses feel more satisfied working in a primary nursing system.

Primary nursing also has an economic advantage: it has been found to be more cost-effective than team nursing in providing high-quality nursing care. Because primary nursing requires registered nurses, it was initially assumed that it would be more expensive than team nursing. However, in terms of salary, actual operating cost, staff development costs, and actual cost per bed, primary nursing was found to be less expensive (Marram, Flynn, Abaravich, & Carey, 1976, pp. 81–85).

Communication is a vital requisite of a smoothly functioning primary nursing system. However, the amount of communication required between primary nurses and the head nurse may be either an advantage or a disadvantage in primary nursing. The head nurse must be knowledgeable about patients currently on the unit, but must also have time to meet newly admitted patients and assign them to primary nurses.

The most obvious disadvantage of primary nursing is the presence of a noncommitted, nonaccountable nurse. The patient's care would suffer because, in this system, there is no one to "pick up after" the nurse. If a nurse previously worked in another type of delivery system in which it was easier to "slack off," she may feel threatened by having to give total care.

An additional disadvantage has to do with associate nurses. Some associate nurses may be unwilling to follow the primary nurse's plan of care. When this happens, quality patient care will not be maintained, and conflicts will arise between primary and associate nurses.

CONCLUSION

Each of the nursing delivery systems has advantages and disadvantages. The nurse-leader must be aware of them and be able to choose the system in which she will feel most comfortable.

Unfortunately, the "real world" does not always conform to the ideal one has in mind. There are many adaptations of team and primary nursing in hospitals, nursing homes, and public health agencies today. The nurse-leader must be on the alert for these, because if she is ready and prepared to function under one system, she will be frustrated and unhappy when she finds a different system in operation.

REFERENCES

Barnard, C. I. *The functions of the executive.* Cambridge, Mass.: Harvard University Press, 1938.

Bullough, V. L., & Bullough, B. *The emergence of modern nursing.* New York: Macmillan, 1969.

Davis, K. *Human behavior at work.* New York: McGraw-Hill, 1977.

Davis, R. C. *The fundamentals of top management.* New York: Harper, 1951.

Fayol, H. *General and industrial management.* London: Pitman, 1949. (Translated from the French edition, 1916.)

Jucius, M. J., Deitzer, B. A., & Schlender, W. E. *Elements of managerial action.* Homewood, Ill.: Irwin, 1973.

Katz, D., & Kahn, R. L. *The social psychology of organizations.* New York: Wiley, 1966.

Lambertson, E. *Nursing team organization and functioning.* New York: Teacher's College, Columbia University, 1953.

Lippitt, G. L. Hospital organization in the post-industrial society. *Hospital Progress,* 1973, *54*(6), 55–64.

Manthey, M., Ciske, K., Robertson, P., & Harris, I. Primary nursing: A return to the concept of "my nurse" and "my patient." *Nursing Forum,* 1970, *9*, 65–83.

Marram, G., Flynn, K., Abaravich, W., & Carey, S. *Cost-effectiveness of primary and team nursing.* Wakefield, Mass.: Contemporary Publishing, 1976.

Roethlisberger, F. J., & Dickson, W. J. *Management and the worker.* Cambridge, Mass.: Harvard University Press, 1939.

Rogers, E. M., & Agarwala-Rogers, R. *Communication in organizations.* New York: Free Press, 1976.

Scott, W. G., & Mitchell, T. R. *Organization theory: A structural and behavioral analysis.* Homewood, Ill.: Irwin & Dorsey, 1972.

Sexton, W. P. (Ed.). *Organization theories.* Columbus, Ohio: Charles E. Merrill, 1970.

Taylor, F. W. *Shop management.* New York: Harper, 1911.

Woodward, J. *Industrial organization: Theory and practice.* New York: Oxford University Press, 1965.

ADDITIONAL READINGS

Becker, S. W., & Neuhauser, D. *The efficient organization.* New York: Elsevier, 1975.

Daeffler, R. J. Patients' perception of care under team and primary nursing. *Journal of Nursing Administration*, 1975, *5*(3), 20–26.

Dowling, W. F. (Ed.). *Organizational dynamics: Making leaders more effective.* New York: AMACOM, 1975.

Hall, R. H. *Organizations: Structure and process.* Englewood Cliffs, N.J.: Prentice-Hall, 1972.

Harrison, E. F. *Management and organizations.* Boston: Houghton Mifflin, 1974.

Longest, B. B., Jr. Institutional politics. *Journal of Nursing Administration*, 1975, *5*(3), 38–41.

March, J. G., & Simon, H. A. *Organizations.* New York: Wiley, 1958.

Marriner, A. Organizational concepts—II. *Supervisor Nurse*, 1977, *8*(10), 37–46.

Miller, P. W. Open minds to new ideas: An injunction for nursing leaders. *Supervisor Nurse*, 1976, *7*(4), 18–22).

Schuldt, S. Supervision and the informal organization. *Journal of Nursing Administration*, 1978, *8*(7), 21–25.

Tannenbaum, A. S. *Control in organizations.* New York: McGraw-Hill, 1968.

Chapter 4

Theories and Styles
of Leadership

The nurse-leader must have an understanding of leadership theories and styles, so that she can select and operationalize those which will be most productive for her in her setting. The purpose of this chapter is to analyze the theories of leadership, and to differentiate among leadership styles. Theories and styles will be applied to contemporary nursing practice in Chapter 5.

DEFINITIONS OF THEORY AND STYLE

When writing about leadership, various authors use theory and style synonymously, or state that the styles of leadership comprise another theory of leadership. However, theory and style are different. Before beginning a discussion of the various theories and styles of leadership, the concepts of theory and style will be defined.

By its very nature, theory is complex and therefore has many definitions. Theory may be defined as a kind of general principle or explanation. Theory is often thought to be a scientifically acceptable general principle that governs practice or is proposed to explain observable facts.

Most significantly, theory represents reality. Concepts found in theories are abstractions that represent real-world phenomena. By specifying relationships among the concepts, a theory explains and predicts actions.

There are four levels of theory or theory building. The first level is concerned with naming or defining and is called *factor-isolating*. This is followed sequentially by the second level, *factor-relating*, which attempts to show relationships among variables. The third level is predictive, specifying the parameters of practice or the timing or direction in a situation. This level is called *situation-relating*, and is closely associated with real-world phenomena. The fourth level is the prescriptive, or *situation-producing* level. In the fourth level, theories from the preceding three levels provide a framework for the desired situation. Calling this fourth level "situation-producing" emphasizes the fact that what practitioners do in the real world does in fact shape and define the practice itself (Dickoff & James, 1975).[1]

Theory, then, serves to specify what type of activity is performed. Theory is the statement of the related factors which define, predict, and prescribe action. In contrast, style refers to how a practice is performed. A style is a manner of acting or a method of performing in a particular situation. Style offers the leader alternative ways of operationalizing a theory of leadership.

Many definitions of leadership have been proposed during the past century. The evolution of leadership theories has followed the pattern of the four levels of theory building. At first, the theories were simplistic, naming the leader and his or her duties, then looking at the differences in leaders and followers to further isolate and relate these variables. Later, the idea of a *situation* or *context* of leadership emerged. Various functions or behaviors for the leader were outlined, and the motivation of the leader's behavior was explored. The concept of style emerged concurrently, giving the leader a choice of methods with which to enact behaviors. Finally, an analysis of variables provided the leader with a way to predict the effectiveness of alternative courses of action. The current and future challenge of theory development in leadership is to arrive at the fourth level, that of "situation-producing," i.e., to refine and expand leadership theory to the prescriptive level.

LEADERSHIP THEORIES

Level I Theory

The Great Man Theory Aristotelian philosophy asserts that some men are born to lead, while others are born to be led. The first recorded theory of leadership, the great man theory, was based on this philosophy.

Reflecting the experience of centuries of rule by monarchs in Europe, it is not surprising that this theory claimed that leaders were born and that leadership was inherited. According to the great man theory, the heir to the throne was expected to possess the abilities that his reign would demand. Being the son of a king somehow ensured such capabilities. This led to the acceptance of intermarriage in the socially elite ruling class in the hope of creating a superior class (Stogdill, 1974, p. 17).

The positive aspect of this theory was the acceptance of the leader-ruler. As long as an heir to the throne was available to assume the responsibilities of his predecessor, no controversy existed.

[1] For a complete understanding of Dickoff and James' theory of theories, see also J. Dickoff, P. James, & E. Wiedenbach. Theory in a practice discipline. *Nursing Research*, 1968, *17*, 415–435.

The negative aspect of the great man theory was that not all those who assumed the role of ruler were capable of leadership. Before this theory lost credibility another theory, the traitist theory, emerged based on great man theory assumptions.

The Traitist Theory The second recognized theory of leadership is the traitist theory. The traitist approach attempted to determine what characteristics a successful leader possessed by studying the leader's personality (Davis, 1977, p. 108). Since it was assumed that leaders were endowed with special qualities that made them superior to their followers, theorists wanted to identify these qualities.

An attempt was made to list qualities hypothesized to be the determinants of successful leadership. The hereditary backgrounds of great rulers were studied to arrive at a list of traits. The supporters of the traitist theory hoped that, once the appropriate qualities were identified, a potential leader could acquire them through study and experience.

While it was found that the leaders often did exceed their followers in intelligence, scholarship, dependability in accepting responsibility, social participation, and socio-economic status, the results of traitist studies were ambiguous. Some leaders had all the described characteristics while others had only one, or none, of them (Stogdill, 1974, p. 62).

The positive aspect of this theory was the effort to define and differentiate between leaders and followers. These attempts to define who the leader "is" did influence later research. Another benefit of the traitist theory was that it asserted that leadership could be learned.

The negative aspect of the traitist theory was that it did not lead to a comprehensive theory of leadership. Although many studies tried to differentiate the characteristics of leaders from those of followers, the effects of leader and follower on each other were not considered. An arena for interaction or a situational context was also seemingly absent in the traitist theory. Some of the studies did note, however, that the qualities demanded of the leader were partially determined by the situation (Stogdill, 1974, p. 62).

Level II Theory

Situational Theory The situational theory of leadership evolved primarily as a reaction to the failure of the traitist approach (Carlisle, 1973, p. 124). A leader, according to this theory, was one who was in a position to institute change when a situation was ready for change (Brown, 1936, p. 331). Leadership was seen as relative to the situation, and in fact was called forth by environmental factors.

The situational theory of leadership attempted to find a flexible approach in which one principle could be used in a variety of settings. The guiding principle in this theory is the situation, or field, which actually determines what the leader does. In situational theory, leadership is the process of influencing a group "in a particular situation, at a given point in time, in a specific set of circumstances" that stimulates the group to achieve objectives with satisfaction (Cribben, 1972, p. 9).

On the positive side, situational theory explored one more variable in the complex phenomena of leadership—the context in which leadership occurs. The main objection to, or negative aspect of situational theory is that a leader does not emerge in every crisis or problem situation. Another problem not resolved by this theory is the uniqueness of situations—even if a leader does emerge due to a situation, this does not ensure effective leadership. Also, being a leader in one situation does not make one a leader in another, so that little direction is provided by this theory. The situational theory was therefore inadequate since an effective leader did not emerge in every situation. Further development of situational theory has occurred, making it a more useful basis for action (for example, Fiedler's contingency model and Hersey and Blanchard's tridimensional leadership effectiveness model, which are discussed later in this chapter).

Interactional Theory If it is neither the leader's personality, nor the situation which determines leadership, then perhaps it is the interaction between these two factors. In addition to the characteristics of the leader and the situation in which he or she functions, the needs and goals of the followers are an important aspect of interactional theory.

Interaction occurs when the behavior of one member causes a change in the behavior of another. This change is in itself a response which stimulates the first member (Bass, 1960, p. 447). The leader stimulates the follower, and the follower, responding, stimulates the leader; this cycle continues and the greater the frequency of interactions, the more effective the group is in moving toward its goal.

In interactional theory, the situation would be classified as having potential for interaction in some degree. Further, leadership is seen as relative to the situation. First, as in situational theory, leadership flourishes in a problem situation. Second, leadership is determined by the goal of the group and is a process of mutual stimulation in which the group's goals as well as the leader's characteristics determine the role of the leader (Gibb, 1947, p. 272).

The interactional theory also attempts to show that, because of a leader's characteristics, he or she is more likely to be chosen by the followers for the leadership role. This supports the earlier view of the traitist theory. Interactional theory, then, is a combination of the situational and traitist theories and shows that leadership is determined by a system of interrelationships.

The positive aspect of the interactional theory is that it made both the traitist and situational theories of leadership usable by relating the characteristics of the leader to the context of the group and the group's goals. It is an important theory in the development of leadership theory because changing a situation is likely to be easier than altering one's personality. The interactional theory supports the belief that anyone can become a leader given an appropriate situation. The only negative aspect of interactional theory is that it does not predict outcomes or prescribe actions that would direct leaders in their role.

STYLES OF LEADERSHIP

The style of leadership used by a leader is dependent on three forces. These forces determine the amount of control a leader will utilize in relating to members of a group. They are found (1) within the leader, (2) within the group members, and (3) within the situation (Tannenbaum, Weschler, & Massarik, 1961, p. 73).

The internal forces, the forces within the leader, include his or her value system, degree of confidence in group members, degree of comfort in the leadership role, and feelings of security in uncertain situations. The leader's value system determines how oriented he or she is to persons or tasks. Values also provide a priority system or framework which allows the leader to assume total responsibility or to delegate responsibility to group members.

Confidence in group members depends upon how much trust has been developed over time with group members. Leaders who feel confidence in group members will consider members' knowledge and competence to be adequate for the task or problems, and will be more inclined to share decision-making responsibility with the group.

Some leaders actively seek control, while others are uncomfortable with total responsibility. The leader who is comfortable in the group and in the leadership role can take control when necessary and share decision-making responsibility whenever possible. Tolerance for ambiguity—the ability to feel secure in uncertain situations—is also an important determinant of the style of leadership the leader will choose (Tannenbaum et al., 1961, p. 74).

The forces within the group members influence the leader's choice of leadership style by clarifying the expectations the group members have of the leader. The leader permits members more freedom when certain conditions exist and less freedom when these same conditions are absent (Tannenbaum et al., 1961, p. 75).

The presence of the following conditions encourages the leader to permit freedom. The group members (1) need independence, (2) show readiness for responsibility, (3) tolerate ambiguity well, (4) are committed to a common goal, (5) are interested in the group task, (6) have the capabilities required to deal with the group task, and (7) expect to share in decision making (Tannenbaum et al., 1961, p. 75). When these conditions are absent, the leader usually retains total control. When these conditions exist, the leader may give up some degree of control to the group members. In doing so, the members' expectations are met and the group becomes more cohesive and more productive (Stogdill, 1974, p. 392).

The amount of freedom given to members and the amount of control given to the leader are also determined by forces within the situation. The traditions and values of the organization in which leaders and members interact are imposed as an unwritten guideline. The size of the organization and its structure certainly determine the amount of interaction possible among the members and with the leader. The degree of confidence members have in the group and the length of affiliation within the group also affect the amount of cooperation within the group. Since working together is essential for group effectiveness, positive past experience with the group encourages further challenge to the group (Tannenbaum et al., 1961, p. 76).

The task or problem confronting the leader determines whether he or she will be able to share decision making with the group. The pressure of time also limits the leader. Groups tend to take longer than one person to arrive at consensus after analyzing the possible solutions. With more time, more input from the group can be sought. These forces within the situation determine the flexibility the leader has to maintain or release control (Tannenbaum et al., 1961, p. 77).

Style is related to the amount of control over or freedom allowed subordinates. The three recognized styles of leadership are *autocratic, democratic,* and *laissez-faire.*

Style can be conceptualized as a range of possibilities along a continuum. The maximum control for the leader with minimum freedom for the group members is the autocratic style. The maximum freedom for the group members with minimum leader control is the laissez-faire style. The range between these two is the democratic style in which the degrees of freedom and control vary (Tannenbaum et al., 1961, p. 69).

Initial research (Lewin, Lippitt, & White, 1939), intended to compare the three styles of leadership, described the leader's behavior in each style. The *autocratic* leader exhibited a consistent behavior pattern—first determining all policies for group members and then detailing methods of goal attainment. The method was shared only in a step-by-step fashion; the leader alone had the overall view. The leader specified both the actions and interactions that would be allowed. Feedback to members was given in the form of personal praise or criticism.

The *democratic* leader encouraged group members to determine their own policies. A leader following this style gave the members an overview of the task and explained all steps toward accomplishment before the group began to work. The leader also allowed the members freedom to choose actions and interactions that would facilitate the work. Feedback was given in a factual and objective manner about the work.

The *laissez-faire* leader gave members complete freedom. Resources for the work were provided, but the leader's participation was limited to answering questions when asked. This type of leader did not give any feedback unless asked.

This research and numerous other studies led to the following conclusions: (1) members of autocratic leader groups became progressively more submissive and demanded attention and approval from the leader; (2) members of democratic leader groups exhibited less tension and hostility (and were more cohesive) than members of autocratic leader groups; and (3) democratic leader groups and autocratic leader groups had about the same productivity, but in comparison, laissez-faire leader groups had lower productivity, satisfaction, and cohesiveness (Stogdill, 1974, pp. 365-370).

Other Styles

The three styles of leadership discussed above can be differentiated further. Some authors propose subcategories along the continuum of possible behaviors. The autocratic style has been called authoritarian, restrictive, and directive. There is agreement that the autocratic leader has a position of centrality allowing him or her to control all information. Some view the autocratic leader as a *paternalistic* figure, having the attitude that "father knows best." This type of leader has a personal relationship with members and provides security and personal rewards to members who comply with his or her direction (Owens, 1976, p. 229).

The autocratic leader has also been conceptualized as an organization person, remaining aloof from members and engaging in one-way communication with the group, telling them what to do. Autocratic leaders may be called *bureaucrats* because their focus on maintaining the organization exceeds their concern for individual workers (O'Donovan, 1975, p. 34).

Another variation of the autocratic style is the *mature autocrat*. Mature autocrats want to have the position of control, yet want the group to feel needed. They are usually highly skilled and persuasive, and sincere about their ideas, and at times invite questions (O'Donovan, 1975, p. 34). The mature autocrat is also known as a *diplomat*, who provides freedom, within strict limits, to group members. This type of leader makes sure that his or her decision is reached, but allows input, so the group remains satisfied that its needs are met (Owens, 1976, p. 230).

The democratic style has also been called participative and egalitarian. The focus of activity in the democratic style is the group. Both the group's task and the individual members are important to the democratic leader. Often the leader will also function as a member of the group during decision-making sessions. The leader may make a tentative decision and test it out with the group, or may present the problem, listen to all the information and alternatives that the group suggests, and then make the decision. These two behaviors allow the group to participate while the leader maintains control over the final outcome (Tannenbaum et al., 1961, pp. 70-71). This is participative, but not egalitarian.

The *collaborative* democratic leader allows the group to arrive at the decision, functioning in a collaborative manner so that free-flowing communication occurs and views are integrated. This style, too, is participative. The *collegial* democratic leader is the egalitarian. While the collaborator performs a supportive team-building function, the colleague focuses more on self-direction by each member within the structure of the organization. Participation is not emphasized to the same degree, and leadership is truly shared equally by every member (Cribben, 1972, pp. 116-119).

The laissez-faire style has been called permissive or free-rein. Often the implication is that the laissez-faire leader abdicates all responsibility and is either absent or not identifiable in the group. The group is given total responsibility but, without any structuring behavior from the leader, the group may be unable to function (Stevens, 1978, p. 129).

Another way of looking at the laissez-faire leader is as a *liberator*. Utilizing the collegial manner, the goals, policies, deadlines, budgets, and all other essential parameters are defined by the group and the leader. The leader then lets the group work independently unless the group requests the leader's participation (Owens, 1976, p. 230).

The laissez-faire style emphasizes the individual rather than the group, leader, or task, and allows open communication among members. The obvious danger in a laissez-faire leader group is the loss of a sense of group unity, which sometimes results in low productivity and little satisfaction (Stogdill, 1974, p. 371).

No one style of leadership is appropriate for every situation encountered by a leader. The leader must choose a style which will best meet the needs of the group members and the goals of the organization, while satisfying the leader's own needs (Carlisle, 1973, pp. 137-138).

In summary, the model in Figure 4-1 attempts to illustrate the range of behaviors possible within the three recognized styles of leadership. Other subcategories are certainly possible, as are combination styles such as the "multicratic" style, which combines the bureaucrat, the mature autocrat, and the democrat to propose an effective range of behaviors for a leader who recognizes that one style alone is not sufficient for every situation (O'Donovan, 1975, pp. 34-35).

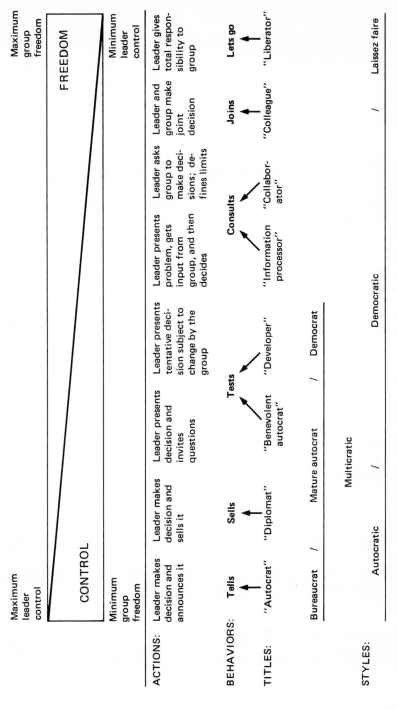

Figure 4–1 A continuum of leadership styles. (*Adapted and expanded from R. Tannenbaum, I. R. Weschler, & F. Massarik. Leadership and organization: A behavioral science approach.*)

LEVEL III THEORIES

The third level in theory building provides theories which go beyond the description level and predict actions. The actions of a leader are predicted in terms of potential effectiveness in the leadership role. Leadership, in third-level theories, is goal-directed behavior. Leadership is the process of influencing an organized group toward goal setting and goal attainment.

Managerial Theory

In the managerial theory of leadership, the leader influences the group by planning, organizing, directing, and controlling the group's behavior. This theory, which is also known as functional or behavioral theory, focuses on the activities of the leader.

Planning refers to the process of determining a course of action in advance of the action (Flippo, 1966, p. 34). Planning is the most basic of all managerial functions, bridging the gap between the present and the desired outcome or goal (Koontz & O'Donnell, 1972, p. 113). *Organizing* is a process of establishing relationships so that energy expenditure is directed toward goal achievement (Flippo, 1966, p. 47). *Directing* is an aspect of the interpersonal process of managing by which members are led to contribute to organizational goals (Koontz & O'Donnell, 1972, p. 499). Directing occurs each time an action is stimulated by the leader (Flippo, 1966, p. 67). *Controlling*, the most necessary behavior, is regulating all activity in accordance with the plan (Flippo, 1966, p. 84).

Many authors specify the activities of the managerial leader using different words, but the framework is basically the same. Planning, organizing, directing, and controlling are the four behaviors or functions which allow the leader to influence the group. Utilizing managerial theory, the leader's influence is focused on moving the group toward the goal.

Zaleznik's Executive Functions

The leader needs a sense of interpersonal competence in order to utilize patterns of influence in a structure of organized human behavior. To enable the leader to maintain the organization, mediate relationships within the environment, and promote creative innovation, three behaviors have been defined. These behaviors, or *executive functions*, are homeostatic, mediative, and proactive (Zaleznik, 1966, p. 172).

The first function, *homeostatic*, is the behavior of the leader that is directed toward assuring the internal stability of the organization (Zaleznik, 1966, p. 173). Ordinarily, little intervention by the leader is needed to maintain the status quo. The homeostatic function, then, is somewhat passive.

The second function, *mediative*, is a more active one than the first. The leader makes a conscious effort to alter the behavior and attitudes of his or her followers. This quest for internal change usually occurs as a response to environmental pressures (Zaleznik, 1966, p. 174).

Instead of being a reaction to environmental pressures, the third function is *proactive*. Proactive behavior induces change by creatively employing organizational resources (Zaleznik, 1966, p. 177).

Table 4-1 Zaleznik's Executive Functions and Leader Actions

	Homeostatic function	Mediative function	Proactive function
Person-oriented leader	Primary action	Secondary action	Avoided action
Fusion-oriented leader	Secondary action	Primary action	Avoided action
Task-oriented leader	Avoided action	Secondary action	Primary action

Source: A. Zaleznik. *Human dilemmas of leadership.* New York: Harper and Row, 1966. © 1966 by Abraham Zaleznik. Reprinted by permission of Harper & Row.

The choice of function or behavior is determined by the leader's orientation to persons or tasks, or to a combination of the two, which Zaleznik calls fusion. The leader's personality helps determine which of the three executive functions will be chosen. As a result, the leader influences followers either to maintain the organization, or to change it in some way.

Although his theory has not been tested, Zaleznik has hypothesized the functional choice and action for each of the three leader orientations, as shown in Table 4-1. Zaleznik believes the person-oriented leader will choose the homeostatic function and avoid the proactive. The task-oriented leader, because of his or her interest in ideas, will choose the proactive and avoid the homeostatic. Finally, the fusion-oriented leader will choose the mediative, but avoid the proactive because of the activity required (Zaleznik, 1966, pp. 191-192).

The personality orientation of the leader is important because it is determined by the leader's goals and needs. Motivation, then, is a key factor underlying Zaleznik's theory. At the core of any theory about influencing persons are assumptions about motivation.

McGregor's Theory X and Theory Y

McGregor (1960) has summarized assumptions about motivation. In his *theory X* he describes the past or traditional view of direction and control. In contrast, in *theory Y*, he proposes an integration of individual goals with organizational goals. X and Y are not opposites; each is a separate philosophy. Both X and Y can be, and frequently are, used. Theory X is the basis of managerial theory; theory Y is the basis for management by objectives.

The assumptions underlying managerial theory, the theory of direction and control that McGregor calls Theory X, are as follows: people dislike work and avoid it whenever they can. Because they dislike and avoid work they must be forced to engage in goal-directed activity. Human beings wish to avoid responsibility, and therefore want to be directed so that they will feel secure (McGregor, 1960, pp. 33-34).

Theory Y proposes a different view of human beings, stating that work is as natural to them as play. Human beings are self-directed and will engage in goal-directed activity by choice, as long as they agree with the goals. The commitment to the goals and the realization of goal achievement is a reward in itself, making direction unnecessary. All individuals are capable of success and in proper conditions will seek responsibility and utilize creativity in problem solving. The creation of conditions that will allow each individual to realize his or her goals is possible (McGregor, 1960, pp. 47–49).

Management by Objectives Through a strategy known as *management by objectives* (MBO), theory Y has been operationalized. Although MBO has been interpreted by some as nothing more than a strategy for management by direction and control, its purpose is to improve job satisfaction by allowing persons to work toward self-actualization while directing their work toward organizational goals (McGregor, 1960, p. 61). MBO substitutes internal or self-control for the managerial external control. It is management by *objectives* rather than management by *control*.

When properly utilized, MBO is a sincere effort to operationalize theory Y. It is a system that integrates the organizational goals of prosperity and growth with the individual's need to contribute to society while developing as a person (Humble, 1973, pp. 4–7).

MBO has been described as the process in which members at two levels of an organization jointly identify goals and designate areas of responsibility (Odiorne, 1965, p. 55). The process consists of a number of interdependent steps.

The first step involves the formulation of objectives by the leader and members together. The objectives are clear, concise, and measurable. The second step is the development of a plan to meet the objectives. The plan is realistic and specific, and provision is made for measurement of performance and achievement in relation to specific target dates. In the final step, any corrective action necessary is taken to accomplish the objectives. The key elements in the process are "goal setting," "action planning," "self-control," and "periodic progress reviews" (Raia, 1974, p. 12).

MBO begins at the highest level of the organization, and is most successful when used at all levels. MBO stresses teamwork. Working together with others instead of competing increases satisfaction and productivity. People compete only with themselves to reach their goals.

There are numerous benefits to the individual and to the organization if MBO is utilized effectively. Each worker is self-directed and not dependent on those above to determine a course of action. The worker self-selects specific goals within the framework of the overall goals of the organization, so that they are congruent. Working independently, the individual may accomplish more and is often more satisfied (Cain & Luchsinger, 1978, p. 38).

Consideration and Initiating Structure

To determine what factors or leader behaviors would have a positive influence on group satisfaction and productivity, numerous investigations have been undertaken. Two behaviors that were found to be important have come to be known as "consideration" and "initiating structure" (Fleishman, 1973, pp. 5–7). *Consideration* is the behavioral dimension of a leader that emphasizes concern for the individual. It includes trust, respect, warmth, and rapport, and encourages communication (Fleishman & Harris, 1962, p. 43).

Initiating structure is the behavioral dimension of a leader that emphasizes concern with the work or goals of the organization. Initiating structure includes defining roles, assigning tasks, planning, and encouraging production in overt ways (Fleishman & Harris, 1962, p. 44).

Research has indicated that group productivity was more closely related to initiating structure, while member satisfaction depended more on consideration than on structure. However, group members did find security in knowing what was expected of them. Group cohesiveness was dependent on both consideration and initiating structure. The most effective leaders were those who utilized both behavioral dimensions, i.e., consideration and initiating structure (Stogdill, 1974, pp. 395-397).

The measurements of consideration and initiating structure were not always so predictable, and some doubt the validity of these behaviors as predictors of effective leadership (Korman, 1966, p. 360). The inconsistencies in the consideration and initiating structure studies suggest that some aspect of the situation may have been inhibiting or modifying the leader-member relationship.

Path-Goal Theory

Path-goal theory attempted to identify the missing situational element by looking at the effect the leader's behavior had on members of the group (Evans, 1970, p. 278). Path-goal theory also specifies conditions in which leader behavior affects member satisfaction (House & Dessler, 1974, p. 54). The degree to which the leader exhibits consideration determines members' perceptions of available rewards, while the degree to which the leader initiates structure determines members' perceptions of paths, or behaviors, which will lead them to their goal (Stogdill, 1974, p. 21).

According to the path-goal theory, the leader initiates structure to show members how their actions will lead to goal attainment and reward. Leaders use consideration to make the path to the goal easier by helping the members remove barriers (Davis, 1977, p. 112). Consideration and initiating structure behaviors increase member motivation and satisfaction to the extent that these behaviors clarify the path to the goal (Evans, 1970, p. 278).

Fiedler's Contingency Model

Utilizing similar variables to arrive at a model of leadership effectiveness, Fiedler (1967) developed the *contingency approach* or contingency theory. Fiedler's model measures leadership effectiveness by looking at group productivity. In this conceptualization, the leader carries the primary responsibility for group task completion. This type of leader may be appointed, elected, or merely identifiable as the emergent leader (Fiedler, 1967, pp. 8-9). Leadership is defined as:

> . . . an interpersonal relation in which power and influence are unevenly distributed so that one person is able to direct and control the actions and behaviors of others to a greater extent than they direct and control his (Fiedler, 1967, p. 11).

Since leadership is a relationship based on power and influence, situations are classified on the basis of the amount of power and influence given to the leader. The measure of power and influence in a situation depends on three variables which, in combination, yield a favorable or unfavorable situation for the leader.

The first factor or variable is leader-member relationships. The assumption that the relationship between the leader and the group members is the single most important variable determining the leader's power and influence is well supported in the literature (Fiedler & Chemers, 1974, pp. 64–65). The degree of acceptance of the leader by the group members determines whether leader-member relationships are classified as good or poor.

The second factor utilized to determine situational favorableness is task structure. A routine, predictable task is said to be structured, while tasks requiring analysis of a variety of possibilities are said to be unstructured.

The third factor, position power, refers to the leader's place within the organization and the amount of authority given to the leader because he or she *is* a leader. Position power may be strong or weak; it does not reflect the strength of the individual leader's personality; rather it measures the leader's status in the organization.

According to Fiedler, these three factors produce eight different situations which are ranked from "most favorable" to "least favorable." Each possible situation is numbered and termed a cell. Cell 1 is the most favorable situation, cell 8 the least favorable.

In Fiedler's initial work, his predictions were as follows: cells 1, 2, 3, and 8 are the very favorable and very unfavorable situations; therefore, a task-centered, controlling behavior will be more effective for the leader. Cells 4, 5, 6, and 7 are intermediate situations; therefore, the permissive, relationship-centered approach will be more effective for the leader (Fiedler, 1967, p. 147). These situations are illustrated in Table 4–2.

More recently, however, Fiedler has determined that only two of the eight cells (4 and 5) represent a situation of intermediate or moderate favorableness requiring a permissive or relationship-oriented approach. He now predicts that, while cells 1, 2, 3, and 8 require a more controlling or task-oriented approach, there is little or no difference in permissive and controlling behavior in cells 6 and 7, which he now classifies as unfavorable to the leader (Fiedler, 1973, p. 28). These situations are illustrated in Table 4–3.

The validity of the contingency model is well supported by research. Although only three variables are analyzed to determine the degree of situational favorableness, these were considered to encompass the most significant factors of the situation (Chemers & Rice, 1974, p. 123).

Although Fiedler's model is predictive and is based on much research, only two conclusions are specified. These conclusions are: (1) task-oriented leaders tend to perform best in groups where the situation is either very favorable or very unfavorable; and (2) relationship-oriented leaders tend to perform best in situations of moderate or intermediate favorableness. No rating is given to the opposite dimension. In other words, a highly task-oriented leader has an unknown relationship orientation, which could be high or low. In fact, any combination of the two orientations is possible (Hersey & Blanchard, 1977, p. 102).

Table 4-2 Fiedler's Contingency Table (1967)

Cell	Leader-member relationship	Structure	Position power	Situation rating	Preferred behavior
1	Good	Structured	Strong	Very favorable	Controlling
2	Good	Structured	Weak	Very favorable	Controlling
3	Good	Unstructured	Strong	Very favorable	Controlling
4	Good	Unstructured	Weak	Intermediate favorableness	Permissive
5	Poor	Structured	Strong	Intermediate favorableness	Permissive
6	Poor	Structured	Weak	Intermediate favorableness	Permissive
7	Poor	Unstructured	Strong	Intermediate favorableness	Permissive
8	Poor	Unstructured	Weak	Very unfavorable	Controlling

Source: F. E. Fiedler. *A theory of leadership effectiveness.* New York: McGraw-Hill, 1967. Used by permission.

Table 4-3 Fiedler's Contingency Table (1973)

Cell	Leader-member relationship	Structure	Position power	Situation rating	Preferred behavior
1	Good	Structured	Strong	Favorable	Controlling
2	Good	Structured	Weak	Favorable	Controlling
3	Good	Unstructured	Strong	Favorable	Controlling
4	Good	Unstructured	Weak	Moderately favorable	Permissive
5	Poor	Structured	Strong	Moderately favorable	Permissive
6	Poor	Structured	Weak	Unfavorable	
7	Poor	Unstructured	Strong	Unfavorable	
8	Poor	Unstructured	Weak	Unfavorable	Controlling

Source: F. E. Fiedler. The trouble with leadership training is that it doesn't train leaders. *Psychology Today*, 1973, *6*(9), 23-30, 92.

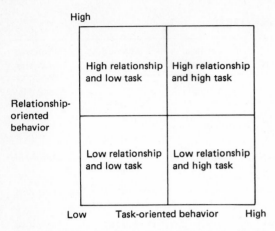

High

High relationship | High relationship
and low task | and high task

Relationship-
oriented
behavior

Low relationship | Low relationship
and low task | and high task

Low   Task-oriented behavior   High

Figure 4-2 The four basic leadership styles used with the tridimensional leadership effectiveness model. (From P. Hersey & K. H. Blanchard. *Management of organizational behavior: Utilizing human resources, 3d ed.* © 1977. Adapted by permission of Prentice-Hall, Englewood Cliffs, N.J.)

Tridimensional Leadership Effectiveness Model

Based on this analysis of Fiedler's theory and on the consideration and initiating structure theories, another way of looking at leadership has been proposed by Hersey and Blanchard. According to these writers, no one leadership behavior or style is effective in every situation. The forces within the leader, the group members, and the situation determine which leadership style a leader uses. Situational favorableness determines the effectiveness of leader behavior. When these factors are combined, a new theory of leadership, the *tridimensional leadership effectiveness model*, emerges.

This theory attempts to integrate leader behavior with situational dimensions. It defines leadership style as the behavior pattern that a leader exhibits "when attempting to influence the activities of others as perceived by those others" (Hersey & Blanchard, 1977, p. 103). The model comprises four basic leadership styles, which can be illustrated in a quadrant system. The four styles are combinations of relationship-oriented and task-oriented behavior (see Figure 4-2).

Hersey and Blanchard define task behavior as organizing and defining member roles and directing activities. Task behaviors are clearly production-oriented. Relationship behavior is person-oriented and consists in facilitating, supporting, and maintaining personal relationships through open communication (Hersey & Blanchard, 1977, p. 104).

To the task and relationship behavioral dimensions (previously defined as initiating structure and consideration) an effectiveness dimension has been added. Effectiveness depends on appropriateness to the situation and is conceptualized on a continuum from effective to ineffective. The four basic styles may be effective or ineffective depending on the action's appropriateness for the situation in the view of group members. The relationship between the behavioral dimensions and the effectiveness dimensions is illustrated in Figure 4-3.

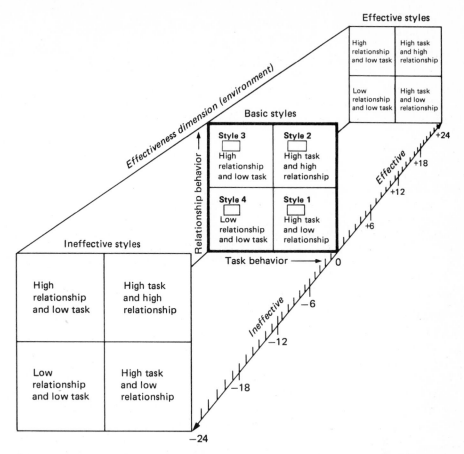

Figure 4-3 Tridimensional leadership effectiveness model: Relationship between behavioral and effectiveness dimensions. *(From P. Hersey and K. H. Blanchard. Management of organizational behavior: Utilizing human resources. Englewood Cliffs, N.J.: Prentice-Hall, 1977. Used by permission of Dr. Joseph W. Keilty, Center for Leadership Studies, Escondido, Calif.)*

For example, a low-relationship, low-task behavior could be viewed by members as appropriately delegating to them the tasks that must be done. In contrast, this same behavior could be viewed as placing all responsibility for the task on the members while the leader avoids responsibility. Any action, therefore, can be considered effective or ineffective depending on how it is perceived by the members.

In order to measure leadership style, Hersey and Blanchard have developed an instrument called Leader Effectiveness and Adaptability Description or LEAD. It is available in two forms—the LEAD-self and the LEAD-other.[2] These tools measure

[2] The LEAD tool and complete instructions for scoring appeared in P. Hersey, K. H. Blanchard, and E. L. LaMonica. A look at your supervisory style. *Supervisor Nurse*, 1976, 7(6), 27–40; as well as in P. Hersey and K. H. Blanchard. *Management of organizational behavior: Utilizing human resources.* Englewood Cliffs, N.J.: Prentice-Hall, 1977.

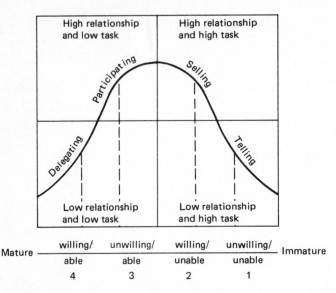

style, style range or flexibility, and style adaptability or effectiveness. By completing the LEAD-self, the leader's perception of his or her own style is identified. The LEAD-other, completed by members, shows their perceptions of the leader's style. Simple numerical calculations from the same tool also measure range and adaptability. Range and adaptability are important because the more flexible a leader can allow him- or herself to be, the more likely the leader is to be effective in any situation.

Even without the LEAD instruments, certain predictions are possible. Looking at members' willingness or motivation in relation to a given task, in addition to their ability or competence, gives an indication of maturity. This maturity factor refers to psychological maturity as well as job maturity. The maturity factor is conceptualized in a separate straight-line continuum placed directly below the four quadrants in Figure 4-4.

The four classifications from lowest to highest maturity are: (1) the member is neither willing nor able to accept this responsibility; (2) the member is willing but unable to accept this responsibility; (3) the member is unwilling but able to accept this responsibility; and (4) the member is both willing and able to accept this responsibility (Hersey & Blanchard, 1977, p. 162).

After deciding which level of maturity is represented by the members, an appropriate style may be chosen. Hersey and Blanchard have determined through research that a curvilinear relationship exists within the quadrants and have given each part of this relational line a style. The high-task, low-relationship quadrant style is called "telling." The high-task, high-relationship quadrant style is called "selling." The low-task, high-relationship quadrant style is "participating." The low-task, low-relationship quadrant style is called "delegating" (Hersey & Blanchard, 1977, p. 169).

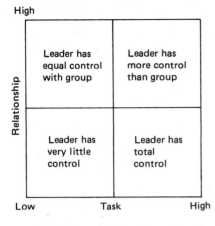

Figure 4-5 Leader and group control in the tridimensional leadership effectiveness model. *(From P. Hersey and K. H. Blanchard. Management of organizational behavior: Utilizing human resources, 3d ed. © 1977. Adapted by permission of Prentice-Hall, Englewood Cliffs, N.J.)*

Members with the lowest level of maturity can be effectively led by using the telling style. Members with the second lowest level of maturity respond better to the selling style. For members in the third level of maturity, participating is the most effective style. Delegating, or allowing a maximum amount of freedom, is most effective for members with the highest level of maturity (Hersey & Blanchard, 1977, p. 170). The relationships between style and maturity are depicted in Figure 4-4.

Other predictions from this model that should help the leader become more effective are: (1) when performance in the group increases, the leader style should shift to the left on the curvilinear line (refer to Figure 4-4); and (2) when performance declines, the leader should shift to the right. These predictions are based on the maturity of the group as reflected in their actual performance (Hersey & Blanchard, 1977, p. 186).

In looking at the amount of leader control and member control, the four quadrants may be compared to the continuum of leadership styles (see Figure 4-1). The leader has greatest control in the high-task, low-relationship quadrant, and least control in the low-task, low-relationship quadrant (Hersey & Blanchard, 1977, p. 217). This is represented in Figure 4-5.

To sum up, the leader has a variety of styles of leadership from which to select. By analyzing the situational variables including leader, members, and environment (situation), an effective style can be predicted.

SUMMARY

Several theories of leadership have been developed which may be useful to the nurse-leader. First-level theories answer the question, "Who is a leader?" Second-level theories and the styles of leadership tell what the leader does or can do. Third-level theories indicate the consequences or possible outcomes of selected leader action. A fourth-level theory of leadership would indicate how a situation should be structured to maximize leadership effectiveness. Chapter 5 will present a framework which may be used by the nurse-leader to develop and operationalize a situation-producing, fourth-level theory.

REFERENCES

Bass, B. M. *Leadership, psychology, and organizational behavior.* New York: Harper, 1960.

Brown, J. F. *Psychology and the social order.* New York: McGraw-Hill, 1936.

Cain, C., & Luchsinger, V. Management by objectives: Application to nursing. *Journal of Nursing Administration,* 1978, *8*(1), 35–38.

Carlisle, H. M. *Situational management: A contingency approach to leadership.* New York: AMACOM, 1973.

Chemers, M. M., & Rice, R. W. A theoretical and empirical examination of Fiedler's contingency model of leadership effectiveness. In J. G. Hunt & L. L. Larson (Eds.), *Contingency approaches to leadership.* Carbondale: Southern Illinois University Press, 1974.

Cribben, J. J. *Effective managerial leadership.* New York: American Management Association, 1972.

Davis, K. *Human behavior at work.* New York: McGraw-Hill, 1977.

Dickoff, J., & James, P. Theory development in nursing. In P. J. Verhonick (Ed.), *Nursing Research I.* Boston: Little, Brown, 1975.

Evans, M. G. The effects of supervisory behavior on the path-goal relationship. *Organizational Behavior and Human Performance,* 1970, *5*, 277–298.

Fiedler, F. E. *A theory of leadership effectiveness.* New York: McGraw-Hill, 1967.

Fiedler, F. E. The trouble with leadership training is that it doesn't train leaders. *Psychology Today,* 1973, *6*(9), 23–30, 92.

Fiedler, F. E., & Chemers, M. M. *Leadership and effective management.* Glenview, Ill.: Scott, Foresman, 1974.

Fleishman, E. A. Twenty years of consideration and structure. In E. A. Fleishman & J. G. Hunt (Eds.), *Current developments in the study of leadership.* Carbondale: Southern Illinois University Press, 1973.

Fleishman, E. A., & Harris, E. F. Patterns of leadership behavior related to employee grievances and turnover. *Personnel Psychology,* 1962, *15*, 43–56.

Flippo, E. B. *Principles of personnel management.* New York: McGraw-Hill, 1966.

Gibb, C. A. The principles and traits of leadership. *Journal of Abnormal and Social Psychology,* 1947, *42*, 267–284.

Hersey, P., & Blanchard, K. H. *Management of organizational behavior: Utilizing human resources.* Englewood Cliffs, N.J.: Prentice-Hall, 1977.

House, R. J., & Dessler, G. The path-goal theory of leadership: Some *post hoc* and *a priori* tests. In J. G. Hunt & L. L. Larson (Eds.), *Contingency approaches to leadership.* Carbondale: Southern Illinois University Press, 1974.

Humble, J. W. *How to manage by objectives.* New York: AMACOM, 1973.

Koontz, H., & O'Donnell, C. *Principles of management: An analysis of managerial functions.* New York: McGraw-Hill, 1972.

Korman, A. K. "Consideration," "initiating structure," and organizational criteria— a review. *Personnel Psychology,* 1966, *19*, 349–361.

Lewin, K., Lippitt, R., & White, R. K. Patterns of aggressive behavior in experimentally created "social climates." *Journal of Social Psychology,* 1939, *10*, 271–299.

McGregor, D. *The human side of enterprise.* New York: McGraw-Hill, 1960.

Odiorne, G. S. *Management by objectives.* New York: Pitman, 1965.

O'Donovan, T. R. Leadership dynamics. *Journal of Nursing Administration,* 1975, *5*(7), 32–35.

Owens, J. The uses of leadership theory. In H. G. Hicks & J. D. Powell (Eds.), *Management, organizations, and human resources.* New York: McGraw-Hill, 1976.

Raia, A. P. *Managing by objectives.* Glenview, Ill.: Scott, Foresman, 1974.

Stevens, W. F. *Management and leadership in nursing.* New York: McGraw-Hill, 1978.

Stogdill, R. N. *Handbook of leadership: A survey of theory and research.* New York: Free Press, 1974.

Tannenbaum, R., Weschler, I. R., & Massarik, F. *Leadership and organization: A behavioral science approach.* New York: McGraw-Hill, 1961.

Zaleznik, A. *Human dilemmas of leadership.* New York: Harper & Row, 1966.

ADDITIONAL READINGS

Barnard, C. I. *The functions of the executive.* Cambridge, Mass.: Harvard University Press, 1938.

Drucker, P. F. *Management.* New York: Harper & Row, 1974.

Fine, R. B. Application of leadership theory. *Nursing Clinics of North America,* 1978, *13,* 139–153.

Gouldner, A. W. (Ed.). *Studies in leadership.* New York: Russell & Russell, 1950.

Guest, R. H., Hersey, P., & Blanchard, K. H. *Organizational change through effective leadership.* Englewood Cliffs, N.J.: Prentice-Hall, 1977.

Hemphill, J. K. *Situational factors in leadership.* Columbus: Ohio State University, 1949.

Hersey, P., Blanchard, K. H., & La Monica, E. A look at your supervisory style. *Supervisor Nurse,* 1976, *7*(6), 27–40.

Hersey, P., Blanchard, K. H., & La Monica, E. A situational approach to supervision: Leadership theory and the supervising nurse. *Supervisor Nurse,* 1976, *7*(5), 17–22.

House, R. J. A path-goal theory of leader effectiveness. In E. A. Fleishman & J. G. Hunt (Eds.), *Contingency approaches to leadership.* Carbondale: Southern Illinois University Press, 1973.

Lewin, K. *Field theory in social science.* New York: Harper, 1951.

Marriner, A. Theories of leadership. *Nursing Leadership,* 1978, *1*(3), 13–17.

Moloney, M. M. *Leadership in nursing.* St. Louis: Mosby, 1979.

Yura, H., Ozimek, D., & Walsh, M. B. *Nursing leadership: Theory and process.* New York: Appleton-Century-Crofts, 1976.

Chapter 5

Components
of Nursing Leadership

Nursing leadership is a multidimensional process that depends upon the relationship
between a nurse-leader and a group, the setting or organization of the interaction,
and the theory of leadership chosen by the nurse-leader. These three components
have been considered as separate entities in the preceding chapters. The purpose of
this chapter is to explore the three components as a unified whole that provides
direction to the nurse-leader.

Every leader must consider each of the three components. Many similarities
exist in all leadership situations, yet the uniqueness of a particular combination of
components cannot be overlooked. The three components are represented in Figure
5-1. Each circle represents the "all possible," all possible combinations of leaders
and groups, all possible settings, and all possible theories of leadership. The overlapping of the circles represents one combination of a particular leader and group,
in a specific setting, with a selected theory or theories.

Every nurse-leader has a group, a setting, and a choice of leadership theory.
By analyzing these three components in relation to each other, the nurse-leader
can determine the behaviors that will enable her to assist her group in goal setting
and goal attainment. In other words, the combination of the three components provides the nurse-leader with a framework from which she can develop her own theory
of leadership.

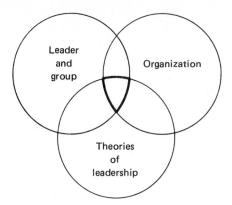

Figure 5-1   Components of nursing leadership.

THE LEADER AND THE GROUP

Nursing leadership is defined as a multidimensional process because the learned and inherited characteristics of the leader are combined with the situational, interactional, and goal-directed dimensions of the first three levels of leadership theory. The learned characteristics of the nurse-leader were identified in Chapter 2 as four attributes: awareness, assertiveness, accountability, and advocacy. The development of these characteristics, or attributes, is an ongoing process, which helps the nurse-leader clarify who she is as a leader.

Another important consideration is the composition of the leader's group. Nurse-leaders have groups with two types of followers—clients of the health care organization (those who seek care) and other members of the health care team (those who give care).

Who the individual followers are as persons becomes an important consideration for the nurse-leader who interacts with the group. The nurse-leader is responsible for coordinating all activities of the group so that each individual follower's needs are met.

The interaction between the nurse-leader and an individual client is a specific type of relationship, often called a *therapeutic relationship*. Specific activities occur within a therapeutic relationship. Often the client seeking care is placed in a dependent position within the health care organization. The nurse-leader seeks to restore the client's independence by engaging in an interdependent relationship with the client until he or she is ready to return to independent functioning.

The interaction between the nurse-leader and another member of the health care organization is also a specific type of relationship, ideally a *collaborative relationship*. Care givers work toward a common goal—the health of their clients. Together the members of the health care organization meet the client. The nurse-leader strives to make this meeting meaningful to the client by collaborating and consulting with health team members involved in that client's care.

Essentially, the nurse-leader is the coordinator of communication. She creates a situation in which therapeutic relationships with clients and collaborative relationships among health team members are possible. By coordinating communication, the nurse-leader assists health team members to achieve the goal of returning clients to independent functioning.

THE ORGANIZATION

The organization is the setting for leader-follower interactions. The philosophy, policies, procedures, and purposes of the organization determine the behaviors that are possible and acceptable for leaders and followers within the organization boundaries. Health care organizations share a common goal: to promote, maintain, and restore the health of clients.

A specific organization may define "client" as an individual person, or as a family, a neighborhood, school, or community. From the organization's definition of whom the client is, specific courses of action are derived.

Individual organizations may also focus efforts on a specific aspect of health care. For example, a rehabilitation institute may focus on restoration of health and have few activities planned for health promotion through prevention. A community health agency may focus its efforts on health promotion, conducting screening programs and providing instruction. Nurse-leaders in a specific setting plan actions that are consistent with the overall purpose and goals of the organization.

Leadership has been defined previously as a process that is used to move a group toward goal setting and goal attainment. This definition is not only compatible with the definition of nursing leadership, it is also an essential component of nursing leadership. This process of goal setting becomes more specific in individual nurse-leader and follower situations in a particular organization.

Deciding upon goals requires the involvement of both the nurse-leader and the followers who participate in the relationship, whether it is therapeutic, collaborative, or both. The amount of involvement possible in such relationships will be determined in part by the persons engaged in the relationship. For example, the developmental level of the client influences the degree to which he or she is able to relate to other persons and to be independent. Also, the personal philosophy of the nurse-leader influences the way in which she relates to others.

The type of organization will also be a determinant. Fewer opportunities for communication and consultation exist in tall organizations. A flat, decentralized organization is designed to foster communication and consultation. Since followers are more likely to be satisfied when they are frequently consulted, the nurse-leader in a tall organization must make greater efforts to create an environment in which dialogue can occur.

THEORIES OF LEADERSHIP

When choosing a theory or theories of leadership to operationalize, it is important for the nurse-leader to analyze the theories critically in light of the goals of the health care organization. It is important to remember that research to judge the effectiveness of theories of leadership has been conducted in a variety of organizations, each with a different goal, and not just in health care organizations.

As nurse-leaders put leadership theories into practice within health care organizations, studies should be conducted to determine the effectiveness of these theories. It will be useful to the development of nursing theory to ascertain which theory or theories foster the goals of health care organizations.

Several theories and styles of leadership were presented in Chapter 4, any of which may be useful to the nurse-leader. The first-level theories have very limited application to nursing, but could be used in combination with other theories. A nurse-leader who chooses a role model, and then tries to act as that person does, may be using the traitist theory. A nurse-leader who identifies herself as a nurse at the scene of an automobile accident may become the situational leader because she could be the most knowledgeable person there at the time.

In the case method and in primary nursing, the nurse-leader spends most of her time in direct contact with clients. Therefore, considering her clients as followers, she might use the interactional theory or, possibly, a third-level theory such as Fiedler's contingency model or the tridimensional leadership effectiveness model.

If the nurse-leader chooses to use the Fiedler contingency model, she first assesses the quality of her relationship with her client. She then determines the amount of power she has in this situation. The task she wishes the client to accomplish is considered next. Once this analysis has been made, she can determine the amount of direction or permissiveness she should use with this client by referring to Table 4-3.

If the nurse-leader decides to use the tridimensional leadership effectiveness model, she must first analyze the maturity of her client. Maturity in this model refers to the client's willingness to engage in the task, and the client's ability to do so successfully. The degree of maturity exhibited by the client determines the behavior of the nurse-leader, as shown in Figure 4-4.

The nurse-leader who is a team leader might choose managerial theory since her leadership role will involve directing team members. The team leader has the responsibility to plan and organize the work of the team. The strategy of organizing presented in Chapter 6 will be useful to nurse-leaders who are team leaders.

Managerial theory is also well suited to the needs of the nurse-leader employed in a setting in which the functional method of organization is used. In such a situation, the nurse-leader is often the only professional nurse involved in the care of several clients; therefore she must structure the situation so that all essential tasks are accomplished efficiently and effectively. Organizing is an important strategy in the functional method.

If a nurse-leader wishes to use either Zaleznik's theory or McGregor's theory, she must examine her own philosophy to determine if her assumptions are compatible with the assumptions that underlie these theories. Management by objectives is not ordinarily the choice of an individual nurse-leader. This method is generally used by nurse-leaders in organizations that operate under the MBO plan.

Although any leadership theory may be used in any setting, none of the existing theories explain specifically how a nurse-leader can promote, maintain, and restore clients' health, or engage in a therapeutic relationship. But the theories do provide a framework for relating to other members of the health care organization. The nurse-leader is challenged to determine the behaviors that will promote, maintain, and restore health.

STRATEGIES FOR NURSING LEADERSHIP

Nursing process is the strategy most often employed by nurse-leaders to set and attain goals. Additional strategies exist that will enable nurse-leaders to move a group toward goal setting and goal attainment. These strategies, which will be discussed in subsequent chapters, are organizing, teaching-learning, decision making, changing, managing conflict, and evaluating.

These strategies are useful processes which may enhance the nurse-leader's effectiveness as leader. In fact, since they indicate behaviors that can be used to move a group toward goal attainment, the strategies themselves are part of a theory of nursing leadership.

ADDITIONAL READINGS

Bailey, J. T., & Claus, K. E. Preparing nurse leaders for the world of tomorrow. *Nursing Leadership,* 1978, *1*(1), 19–28.

Chater, S. S. A conceptual framework for curriculum development. *Nursing Outlook,* 1975, *23*, 428–433.

Corona, D. F. Followership: The indispensable corollary to leadership. *Nursing Leadership,* 1979, *2*(2), 5–8.

Diamond, H. Patterns of leadership. *Image,* 1979, *11*, 42–44.

Fuller, S. Humanistic leadership in a pragmatic age. *Nursing Outlook,* 1979, *27*, 770–773.

McNally, J. M. Leadership—the needed component. *Nursing Leadership,* 1979, *2*(3), 6–12.

Tyndall, A. Situational leadership theory. *Nursing Leadership,* 1979, *2*(2), 25–29.

Chapter 6

The Nurse-Leader
and the Process
of Organizing

Organizing is a process used by the nurse-leader as part of the leadership process. Organizing may be defined as the arranging of component parts into a functioning whole. The purpose of organizing is to coordinate activities so that a goal can be achieved. Organizing, then, is a means to an end, not an end in itself.

The terms "planning" and "organizing" are often used synonymously. For example, organizing is not considered a step in the nursing process; however, planning is the second step. In the managerial process (i.e., managerial theory of leadership) planning is considered the first step and organizing, the second.

In the managerial process, planning is the determination of what is to be accomplished, and organizing, the determination of how it will be accomplished. However, most authors still describe the two processes with considerable overlap.

In the nursing process, planning includes writing objectives, setting priorities, and determining activities to meet the objectives (Yura & Walsh, 1978, p. 116). Thus, organizing may be considered part of planning, even though it is not specifically identified. Planning, and thus organizing, may be viewed broadly as being part of all processes, including the leadership process. Thus, planning and organizing may be said to answer the what, why, how, who, when, and where questions about specific activities.

The process of organizing is used by the effective nurse-leader with every group she leads, regardless of its size. It is used for example, by the nurse-leader who, as a director of nursing, establishes a nursing service in a hospital, nursing home, school, or public health agency. It is used by nurse-leaders who, as head nurses or team leaders, make patient care assignments to other nursing personnel. It is also used by the nurse-leader who, as a primary nurse or staff nurse, gives direct care to patients.

There are six steps in the organizing process. They are as follows:

1 Establish overall objectives
2 Formulate derivative objectives, policies, and plans
3 Identify and classify activities necessary to accomplish the objectives
4 Group the activities in light of the human and material resources available and the best way of using them
5 Delegate to the head of each group the authority necessary to perform the activities
6 Tie the groups together horizontally and vertically, through authority relationships, and information systems (Koontz & O'Donnell, 1976, p. 279)

An explanation of the steps and their application to nursing is the focus of this chapter.

ESTABLISH OBJECTIVES

The first step in the process of organizing is to establish overall objectives. Objectives are explicit, concise statements of what is to be accomplished. They provide direction for selecting materials and methods to achieve the desired goal (Mager, 1962, p. 13). Behavioral objectives can be measured through observable performance. Overall objectives are usually broad and give a general idea of what is to be accomplished.

Five criteria for sound objectives have been established (Jucius, Deitzer, & Schlender, 1973, pp. 167-168). First, the objective must be *acceptable* to both the leader and the group who will be involved in achieving it—they must agree that it is worthy of their efforts. All members of the group should see the objective as related to the purpose of the group.

Second, the objective must be *attainable* within a reasonable period of time, that is, it must be realistic. If an objective is acceptable, but too "lofty" for speedy achievement, it should be broken down into several, more short-term objectives. "Quadriplegic patients will be able to feed themselves before they are discharged" is an acceptable objective, but it may take a considerable amount of time to achieve. It might be better to specify several smaller objectives, such as, "quadriplegic patients will state that they wish to feed themselves," "quadriplegic patients will explain the use of assistive aids for eating," and "quadriplegic patients will feed themselves with the use of assistive aids."

Third, the objective must be *motivational*, that is, it should be stated in such a way that it causes the group to want to strive toward reaching it. When the nurse-leader collaborates with group members in establishing objectives, members' ideas should be included, so that they will feel a part of the objective. When members have input into the objective, it becomes their own, and they are motivated to achieve it.

Fourth, the objective must be *simple*. It should clearly describe only one behavior.

A good objective is as brief as possible, yet its meaning is clear. Objective A below is too complex and wordy, and has more information than is needed. Objective B is a satisfactory objective, stating the same purpose simply and concisely.

> *Objective A:* Mrs. Day, with assistance from a nursing assistant to carry her IV and push her Gomco, will ambulate safely, and at reasonable speed, to the nursing station, which is 1000 feet from her room, three times every 24 hours, from 8 a.m. to 8 a.m.
>
> *Objective B:* Mrs. Day will walk to the nursing station three times a day.

Finally, the objective must be *communicated* to all persons who are concerned with its achievement. The leader, the group, and their superiors should all know, initially and throughout the process, the goals toward which they are working.

FORMULATE DERIVATIVE OBJECTIVES

There is no clear break between the first and second steps in the organizing process. From the initial overall objectives the nurse-leader has identified, more specific objectives can be written. As stated earlier, good objectives must be easily attainable, and it is for this reason that more specific objectives are established. All objectives must be consistent with the overall objectives of the organization.

Another part of the second step in the organizing process is the recognition of existing policies, procedures, and rules that affect the task and objectives. A policy is a guide to action that provides a standard decision for recurring problems of a similar nature (Jucius et al., 1973, p. 173). Policies are usually made by top-level administrators, and they apply throughout the organization. Policies aid in keeping activities in line with the overall objectives of the organization. For example, "all patients being discharged must go to the door in a wheelchair" is a policy to aid in meeting the overall goal, "patients will not fall in the hospital."

Most health care institutions have procedure manuals. Procedures describe the step-by-step approach to the completion of a particular task. Since procedures may vary from institution to institution, the nurse-leader must be familiar with the procedures used in her setting. The brands of products used by an institution often determine the procedure to be used.

In addition to general policies and procedures, an individual nursing unit may have rules that govern specific actions in that unit only. A rule on one nursing unit may be: "each nurse provides her own patients with fresh ice water," and on another unit: "nursing assistants pass fresh ice water to all patients every day, about 10:30 a.m."

The nurse-leader must be cognizant of the institutional objectives, policies, and procedures, as well as the individual nursing unit rules, so that the objectives she establishes can be met. If a policy states that a registered nurse must discharge all patients, an objective cannot provide for nursing assistants or volunteers to discharge patients.

IDENTIFY AND CLASSIFY ACTIVITIES

The next step in the process of organizing is to identify and classify the activities that are necessary to achieve the objectives. If the written objectives are very specific, the required activities will be obvious.

The activities that a primary nurse will have to perform to provide care for a group of five patients include such things as patient teaching, giving medications and treatments, bathing patients, and making beds. The activities that a team leader with a group of fifteen patients and three staff members must perform include, in addition to the above, such things as planning and leading a team conference, supervising team members, and admitting patients.

Certain activities, such as passing meal trays, must be done every day, and are subject to very little change. Others, such as treatments and medications, vary considerably from day to day. The nurse-leader must remember to identify the non-variable activities as well as the variable ones.

The nurse-leader not only determines what activities must be performed, but also when, where, how, and why they must be done. Some medications may be given every hour, some as needed, and some just once a shift. Other activities may be performed only once in 24 hours (e.g., baths), or once a month (e.g., comprehensive evaluation of rehabilitation clients). If advance scheduling is necessary (e.g., for x-ray), the scheduling itself becomes another activity for the nurse-leader.

Some activities will be done in the patient's room or home; others may be done at a clinic or elsewhere. If transportation is required, arranging for it must also be included in the activities.

It is important for the nurse-leader to know *how* activities are done. If one patient does her colostomy irrigation with one brand of apparatus and another patient uses a different brand, the minor differences may be important. If a special procedure has been modified, or adapted, for a particular patient, the "how" is very significant.

The nurse-leader should also know *why* activities are done. If vital signs were ordered every hour for a patient who appears to be recovering normally from surgery, the nurse-leader should know the reason, since it may affect her organization plan. The nurse-leader will also want to explain the reason to her group. In addition, if she knows the physician's routines, she may be able to change the order, assuming there is no current rationale and it is simply an old order that was never changed.

Priority Setting

Once all the activities have been identified, they should be classified, i.e., given priorities by the nurse-leader. Classifying activities according to priority involves making choices about the importance of each activity and deciding the order in which they will be carried out. *Priority setting* is thus defined as determining the relative importance among tasks which must be done, and establishing an order for them. Priorities are established for the entire task (e.g., care of five patients), and also for the activities in the care of each of the five patients.

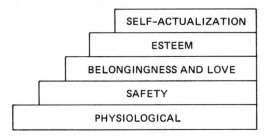

Figure 6–1 Maslow's hierarchy of needs.

The nurse-leader must have a rationale for the way the priorities are established. They should be established based on the nurse-leader's knowledge of the biological and behavioral sciences. In patient care, the importance of one activity over another is most often determined on the basis of how potentially life-threatening a particular situation is for the patient.

Using Theory as a Basis for Priority Setting Two well-known theories can easily be applied as rationale for priority setting. The first is Maslow's (1954) hierarchy of needs. According to this theory, needs are organized hierarchically, and lower-level needs must be met before higher-level needs are considered. Maslow identifies five levels of needs, which are shown in Figure 6–1.

The physiological needs—including hunger, thirst, oxygen, sleep, activity, and elimination—are necessary for survival, and so may be considered the most important or highest-priority needs. Safety needs—which include shelter, clothing, and protection—are also very important for an individual's security and growth. Higher needs are not imperative for life, and consequently will not usually be recognized until the lower needs are met (Maslow, 1954, pp. 147-150). For example, it is more important to be able to breathe than to deal with the reasons for one's depression.

A nurse-leader who uses this theory as the rationale for her priorities will be most concerned with the physiological needs of her clients, and will give them highest priority. In terms of activities, she will place emphasis on those activities necessary for maintenance of life, e.g., assisting with eating (nutrition and hydration needs), or bowel programs (elimination needs).

A second priority for the nurse-leader would be safety needs, such as the need for an orderly, predictable environment. Safety needs are related to protection. The nurse-leader would rate prevention of falls and prevention of skin breakdown as moderate- to high-priority.

Love, esteem, and actualization needs are considered higher-level needs, and have a lower priority than physiological or safety needs. Love needs involve personal relationships and being part of a group. Esteem needs involve a person's need for self-respect and attention. Self-actualization means doing what one is best suited for. The nurse-leader will not neglect these higher-level needs, but they will be given a low priority until the other needs are met.

When lower-level needs have been met, the nurse-leader will be more involved with love, esteem, and/or actualization needs, and may give them high priority. For example, a school nurse is asked to talk with a 16-year-old boy who is doing very poorly in school. She learns that the adolescent comes from a very wealthy family and has all the material things he could want, i.e., his physiological and safety needs are met. However, the boy tells her that he is new in the school and cannot seem to make any friends. The nurse-leader quickly realizes that his love and belongingness needs must be given the highest priority. All five levels of needs are important, and the nurse-leader must be able to determine which are most important to her clients at a particular time so that she can set appropriate priorities.

The second theory that can be used for priority setting is Levine's (1967) conservation principles. According to Levine, nursing intervention is concerned with four conservation principles. While this approach is a holistic one in which, ideally, all four principles are utilized at all times, it can still serve as a guide to priority setting.

The first principle involves *conservation of energy* and stresses the importance of basic life processes. The functional ability of a person is determined by the amount of energy available to that person. Biologically, energy refers to the exchange of nutrients and oxygen. The availability of nutrients and oxygen, as well as the ability to use these resources, is important. The rate at which energy is utilized must also be considered.

For example, a healthy individual may increase the rate of energy consumption by running. If unlimited oxygen and nutrients are available, there is no threat to health, even during prolonged running. If, however, the runner is anemic, an increase in oxygen use could pose a serious threat to health, since oxygen cannot be transported effectively.

The priority at this level would be to increase the amount of usable energy available in order to maintain life. A variety of specific interventions exist to meet this goal. The priority is the maintenance of life by supplying energy for the basic life processes. The first level or core of the person is of the greatest importance.

The second conservation principle is that of *structural integrity*, which stresses the importance of the body as an intact system where structure protects functional processes. Second in priority, therefore, are interventions that maintain an individual's structural integrity.

For example, since the skin serves as a barrier to pathogens in the environment, nursing intervention focuses on maintaining skin integrity. Priority interventions at this level are selected because structural integrity protects the core—the energy or functional process level.

The first and second principles focus on maintaining life at a very basic level, while the remaining two principles focus on a meaningful existence, which can occur only if life is maintained.

The third principle is that of *personal integrity*. This conservation principle stresses the holistic nature of persons, maintaining that the individual is more than structure and energy—the mind and spirit which make the person unique are also essential to meaningful life. Nursing interventions at this level focus on maintaining and strengthening inner resources that sustain the unique self and relieve feelings that interfere with total functioning.

When a child becomes acutely ill, the parent caring for her may feel responsible for the illness. The parent's guilt feelings may interfere with self-image and with child care duties. The priority would be to provide the parent with a realistic perception of the situation, in hopes of diminishing guilt and restoring total functioning.

The fourth conservation principle is concerned with *social integrity*. This principle stresses the importance of the immediate environment for the comfort and safety of the person. Social integrity also includes significant relationships with other people. Priority interventions at this level focus on maintaining a healthy, satisfying environment, including meaningful relationships. Examples of nursing interventions at this level are selecting compatible roommates in a health care facility and providing privacy for each individual.

Levine's conservation principles stress four important components of meaningful human existence. Priorities can be set for nursing interventions by utilizing these principles as a way to check that all important aspects of care have been considered. When it is not possible to carry out activities on all four levels, the highest priority is given to the core, or energy level. Structural, personal, and social integrity then become lower priorities, as shown in Figure 6-2.

Factors Affecting Priority Setting   No matter what theory is used, the priorities that the nurse-leader sets will be affected by a number of practical considerations.

Time   The first of these factors is time. The ability to accurately predict the length of time it will take to complete an activity is extremely useful. This ability allows the nurse-leader to estimate how many activities can be scheduled and also gives flexibility to her plan.

The length of time needed to complete an activity may influence the priority it is given. An activity that takes a long time may be a high priority or a low priority. Bathing a semicomatose patient takes a great deal of time, but the nurse-leader may

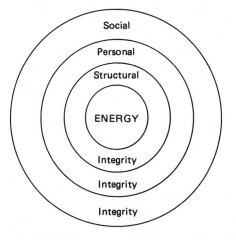

Figure 6-2   Conceptualization of person according to the conservation principles.

give this activity a high priority because the patient needs to be clean and dry, and to be moved around to prevent skin breakdown and contractures. On the other hand, the nurse-leader may give this activity a low priority because she can perform a number of other activities for other patients during the time it would take to give a single patient a bath.

It is possible to organize solely on the basis of time. The nurse-leader determines the activities which must be done, and decides on a time for each. Figures 6–3 and 6–4 show how a team leader and a team member organized their work by time alone.

Figure 6-3   A team leader's organization plan, based on time, for one daytime shift.

Daily work plan

Team leader ___*John*___   Date ___*6-25-80*___

7:00   *get report, prepare assignments*

7:30   *give report to team*

8:00   *pass trays, meds*

8:30   *make rounds*

9:00   *meds*

9:30   ⎫
          assist
10:00 ⎬ *team*

10:30 ⎭

11:00 *lunch*

11:30 *pass trays*

12:00 *meds*

12:30 ✓ *orders*

1:00   *meds*

1:30   *get report from team*

2:00   *make rounds*

2:30   *tape report*

3:00   ✓ *narcotics*

Patient	4	5	6	7	8	9	10	11
12 Mrs. Paul, 62 CVA	Rom		Rom		Rom		Rom back care	I&O
14A Mr. Brown 47 MI				up			back care	I&O
14B Mr. Smith, 52 Ulcer	milk	maalox	milk	maalox	milk	maalox	milk	maalox
17 Miss Grany 22 PID								I&O
21A Mrs. March, 43 GI workup						enema		
21B Mrs. Peters, 36 Asthma	IPPB				IPPB			I&O

Daily work plan — Team member Teresa — Date 6-25-80

Figure 6-4 A team member's organization plan, based on time, for one evening shift.

The nurse-leader who organizes solely by time will probably be very organized, and will have set priorities. However, her priorities are likely to include only those activities that have little variance. It is possible to use a time-card approach to rank important nursing care activities, but the nurse-leader must be careful to remember that priorities must be given to variable activities as well.

Policies, Rules, and Procedures Another factor that affects priority setting is the existence of various policies, rules, and procedures. Policies, rules, and procedures are meant to simplify nursing care, so that a nurse-leader will automatically know what to do in a given situation. Thus, policies may determine the priority of a particular activity.

If a hospital policy says that preoperative medications are given exactly 1 hour before the scheduled time of surgery, giving the medications at the appropriate time becomes a high priority. Another policy might say that all patients must have their baths before going to physical therapy; in that case, giving baths to all the patients the nurse-leader is caring for who have physical therapy is probably a higher priority than giving baths to the other patients.

Experience and Values of the Nurse-Leader The nurse leader's past experience and her value systems have a great effect on the priorities she sets. The nurse-leader will place a high priority on activities that she likes to do, activities that she has learned from in the past, and activities she simply thinks are critical. Her basis may be in knowledge or intuition. She may place low priority on activities that she does not enjoy doing, or on tasks she has never done or is not quite sure how to do.

When a nurse-leader has learned from past experience that it is rarely successful to teach a patient about diet on the day he or she goes home from the hospital, she will make diet teaching a higher priority earlier in the patient's hospital stay. If a school nurse likes to teach sex education, she may automatically make it a high priority; however, if she is uncomfortable teaching sex education, she may give it a low one, or not teach it at all.

Patient's Desires and Preferences The patient's preferences must also influence the priorities that the nurse-leader establishes. What a nurse-leader might call "little things" may be of the utmost importance to the patient—for example, watering the patient's flowers. Some patients have a daily routine that they do not want changed when they enter a hospital or nursing home; for them, it is a high priority.

A client's involvement in priority setting depends on four things: the nature of the health problem, the client's understanding of the situation, the client's desire to be involved (Bower, 1979, p. 238), and the willingness of the nurse-leader to allow that involvement. Some clients and their families want very much to be involved in their care, while others prefer having the nurse-leader do everything for them. Other patients would like to be involved but, because they are too sick, or else do not understand their condition completely, they are unable to participate fully or at all.

A nurse-leader who believes in client involvement in care and priority setting will find ways to teach clients and help them be involved as much as possible. Nurse-leaders who find it easier to set priorities themselves will find ways to avoid client involvement. Neither is the better solution; client involvement depends primarily on the patient's interest and ability.

A new mother who has had a successful vaginal delivery and is delighted with being a parent may wish to be completely involved in her own and her baby's care, and this should be encouraged by the nurse-leader. But a new mother who has had an emergency caesarean section and who was not very happy being pregnant may not be as able or willing to be involved in her own care and that of her baby.

When the patient's desires and the nurse-leader's beliefs about priorities differ, a compromise must be reached. One approach to dealing with such a conflict is to set priorities on the basis of actual and potential problems. In this approach, priorities are arranged on four levels: (1) all problems involved with the life and safety of the client; (2) actual problems the client deems important; (3) actual or potential problems that the nurse-leader believes are important, but that the patient does not recognize; and (4) potential problems the patient deems important (Kron, 1976, p. 118). The nurse-leader can share with the patient this method of arranging the priorities, so that both the patient's and the nurse-leader's wishes can be satisfied.

A 70-year-old man who has had a cerebral vascular accident and is newly admitted to a rehabilitation hospital may have some priorities that differ from the nurse-leader's. If the nurse-leader discusses the actual and potential problem approach with him, together they may set priorities for categories such as (1) assistance with ambulation,

(2) learning to dress, (3) prevention of contractures on his paralyzed side, and (4) getting his home rearranged so that he can go home.

Practicalities of Priority Setting There are several things that the nurse-leader must remember when setting priorities. The first and most important is that priorities change! Literally anything can happen, at any time, that may warrant a change in priorities. Both "routine" events, such as patients being taken to or brought back from surgery, meal trays being early or late, new orders, admissions and discharges of patients, and emergency events, such as a patient falling out of bed or having a cardiac arrest can alter priorities. In setting priorities, the nurse-leader must be cognizant of the fact that she must be flexible.

The nurse-leader must be careful to set priorities each day for *all* the activities in her responsibility. She may not be able to complete them all on a given day or complete them in the way that she wants; however, an activity that has a low priority one day, and is not finished, may become a higher priority the next.

The nurse-leader should write her priorities on paper and carry the list with her. Because she is responsible for a large number of activities, she should not trust her memory. As activities and priorities are completed, the nurse-leader can mark them off her list and/or write notes to herself about important things to remember that she should report to the supervisor, physician, or next-shift nurses. She can also add activities and revise her list if changes occur.

GROUP ACTIVITIES

The fourth step in the process of organizing is to group activities according to the human and material resources available. In nursing language, grouping activities is similar to making assignments. Once all the activities have been identified and given a priority, the nurse-leader must analyze her resources, so that they can be used to best advantage—in terms of time, talents, and economy. The nurse-leader must assess both her group members and the material resources she has at hand or can obtain.

When making assignments, a nurse-leader who is a team leader or charge nurse must be aware of the needs, beliefs, experience, preferences, strengths, and limitations of each group member. The nurse-leader will strive to assign to each member an activity that will provide a new learning opportunity and still be within the ability of the member to perform and to enjoy.

Room placements of patients should be taken into consideration when making assignments, but assignments should be made on the basis of client needs and group member qualifications, *not* on the basis of room numbers. Consideration should be given to avoiding excessive walking for nurses by not assigning them to critical patients on both ends of a long corridor. (A better solution might be to move critical patients closer together and closer to the nurses' station.)

The nurse-leader will want to obtain input from her group members regarding which activities they would like to do. Sometimes this is done informally; the nurse-leader quickly asks each member if there is anything he or she would rather do or not do. The team leader may also discuss preferences more formally with her group in a team meeting at which all the activities are presented and discussed, and the assignments are made with the nurse-leader and group collaborating. The nurse-leader must be sure that each activity is clearly assigned to a specific group member.

The nurse-leader must be aware of the *job descriptions* for each of her group members. A job, or position, description is a formal document, usually prepared by the administration of an organization, which describes the work, and the parameters of the work, for each title within the organization, e.g., head nurse, team leader, licensed practical nurse, or clinical specialist. The nurse-leader cannot assign an activity to a group member that is not within the responsibilities included in that member's job description.

Established priorities and client preferences must be taken into account when making assignments. Because of the priority needs of a client, or of the limited number of group members, a member may have to be assigned to the care of a patient whom she would rather not handle. In this instance the nurse-leader will probably want to work closely with and assist the group member. The nurse-leader must not let the patient's care suffer because the member is less than satisfied with the responsibility.

Material resources must also be considered when grouping activities or making assignments. For example, on a thirty-bed unit at a nursing home, there are ten patients who could have wheelchair showers, but only one wheelchair shower. The nurse-leader must decide how best to use the wheelchair shower to benefit her clients and to best use the time of her group members. In the same nursing home, a priority has been established for teaching another patient about her diet, but all the dietary audio-visual equipment is being used by someone on another unit. The nurse-leader will have to change either the priority or the teaching method.

From these examples it can be seen that available resources affect priority setting. If the desired resources are not available, or will be available only at a later time, then the priorities may need to be revised.

However, priorities should still be set before considering either human or material resources, because the nurse-leader can then tell her superior, on the basis of the available data, that the resources are needed. She may not always get what she wants, e.g., another nurse or more equipment, but at least she has shared the need with her superior, and made it clear why the need exists. The next time she may obtain the resources she needs.

DELEGATION

Once the nurse-leader has arranged the activities in order of priority, with the available resources, she can move to the next step in the organizing process—delegating authority to the group to carry out the activities. Delegation of authority is probably the most important step in organizing.

Delegation is the process of assigning part or all of one person's responsibility to another person or persons. It is something that the nurse-leader *must* do. The purpose of delegation is efficiency; no one person can do all the work that must be done; therefore, some work must be passed on, or delegated, to others. However, it must be remembered that, even when an activity is delegated to someone else, the ultimate responsibility for that activity still belongs to the nurse-leader, i.e., the person who delegated the activity.

Problems with Delegation

Some leaders have difficulty delegating, and this poses two major problems for the organization. First, the leader who does not delegate enough becomes overworked. An overworked leader quickly becomes tired and ineffective and as a result the system may break down.

Second, group members who are not delegated enough responsibility will become bored, lazy, and ineffective. This may also cause system breakdown. It is a common experience in nursing, as elsewhere, that more mistakes are made on slow days than on hectic days.

Group members who have a leader who delegates well benefit in three ways: (1) their sense of responsibility is enhanced; (2) they increase their knowledge; and (3) their job satisfaction is enhanced (Beyers & Phillips, 1979, p. 197). Ultimately the group will be happy, morale good, and production high; therefore the organization is likely to be functioning at its peak.

Leaders have many reasons for not delegating sufficiently. These reasons may be grouped into three categories: the leader's feelings about the activity, the leader's feelings about self, and the leader's feelings about the group.

What a leader believes about an activity affects the decision to delegate it. Some reasons why the leader may not delegate an activity include:

1　It is too difficult an activity for the group.
2　It would take more time to explain the activity to the group than to just do it.
3　The activity can only be performed by a certain type of person.
4　There are legal ramifications involved with the activity.

Many reasons why a leader does not delegate relate to feelings about self. For example:

1　I am responsible for the work anyhow, so I may as well do it.
2　I like to do this activity.
3　It makes me feel good to be able to do the activity alone.
4　I can do the job better than anyone else.
5　I will lose control if I let someone else do it.

The leader's feelings about the group have a great deal to do with how much work is delegated. For example, the leader may feel that

1　Group members cannot be trusted to do the activity correctly.
2　They do not have enough experience or skills to do it.
3　They have enough to do without adding this activity.
4　They will not keep me informed about what is happening.

5 They will want more money if they have to do more work.
6 They might become too good and then want my job.

One of the principal reasons why leaders delegate poorly, or not at all, may be that they simply do not know *how* to delegate.

Delegation may also fail because of the group. There are two main reasons why group members hesitate to accept the authority that has been delegated: they are afraid of failure, and they lack confidence—in themselves and/or in their leader (Jucius et al., 1973, p. 244). These two reasons are closely related.

Many people are afraid to do anything new because they do not trust themselves to do it right; they have little or no self-confidence, and they are afraid of what will happen if they do something wrong. Mistrust of the leader may also cause group members to be skeptical of accepting anything delegated to them. Members will mistrust a leader who makes ambiguous assignments, who plays members against each other, who expects members to cover for the leader's mistakes (Jucius et al., 1973, p. 244), or who does not delegate the needed authority for the assigned task.

How to Improve Delegation

Leaders can do many things to improve delegating skills. First, they should carefully assess feelings about themselves as leaders, about group members, and especially about delegation in general. Once these feelings have been assessed, and the leader consciously wants to delegate effectively, he or she should carefully examine the activities to be delegated.

The leader should define the activity clearly and then share the definition of what is to be done with the person to whom the activity is delegated (Volante, 1974, p. 21). It is exceedingly important to be explicit about *what* is to be done. If the leader and the follower both know exactly what is to be done, neither should fear the delegation process.

The leader can determine with the follower whether or not the leader needs to give directions about how to do the activity. If the leader has thoroughly assessed group members, it should be clear whether a particular member can do the activity, or whether he or she will need help.

It is essential that the nurse-leader also delegate the appropriate authority (power to act) for the activity assigned. A group member cannot function without the needed authority. Both leader and member will know that sufficient authority has been delegated when the member is able to make the necessary decisions about the performance of the assigned activity. The leader *must* delegate authority!

The leader must arrange with the group for feedback about the activities and their accomplishment. When both the leader and group are clear about what the activities are, it will be easy for the group to inform the leader about progress, or lack of it, in completing the work. However, the leader must establish with the entire group, and/or with each individual group member, a specific time and place at which feedback will be given. Progress reports must be obtained because the leader is still responsible for the activity, and will have to account for it to his or her superior.

Finally, the leader should be ready to reward group members for successful assumption of authority (Koontz & O'Donnell, 1976, p. 384) and completion of assigned activities. Group members whose contributions are appreciated by the leader will be better motivated to accept further responsibilities. A simple "thank you" goes a long way.

Giving Report

Every time a nurse-leader asks someone to do something for her, she is delegating a part of her responsibility. For example, if a primary nurse asks a nursing assistant to make a bed for her, she has given the nursing assistant part of her responsibility for the care of a specific patient. When a head nurse divides her unit into three teams, and assigns a team leader and certain staff members to each team, she has delegated her responsibility for the care of all the patients on her unit.

In nursing, delegation is closely tied to giving report. Reports are given by nurse-leaders to their superiors, their peers, and their group members. A report to one's superior is accounting for one's responsibility.

Reporting to one's peers—for example, a change-of-shift report—is both a delegation of responsibility and an accounting of what has been done. Technically, responsibility is only delegated by one's superior, but change-of-shift reports are given to prepare personnel for their responsibility. When an evening nurse reports to a night nurse, she is accounting for what she did, but she is also assisting the night nurse to know what she must do.

A report from a nurse-leader to her group members is truly a delegation of responsibility and authority. When assigning the care of a patient to a group member, the nurse-leader should give the member significant information about the patient, as well as complete information about what the member is to do. The use of a Kardex and/or nursing care plan aids in giving report because a specific format is used, and thus the report for each patient will follow the same pattern. The member will know the type of information that is coming next, and can be more involved in the report. Questions may be asked, so that information is clarified and the nurse-leader and the member have the same expectations.

Certain components may be considered essential when giving a change-of-shift report. The name, room number, and diagnosis of each client must always be given. Sometimes the name of the physician responsible for the care of the patient is also given. The report deals primarily with what happened to the patient during the ending shift. Pertinent information regarding what happened to the patient in the previous one or two shifts should also be reported. Finally, a change-of-shift report should always begin at a specified time, so that staff from both shifts are ready to be involved.

TYING TOGETHER

The final step in the process of organizing is that of coordination. Groups or group members must be placed horizontally and vertically into a framework of authority relationships and information systems in the organizational structure. Again there is no clear break between delegation and this step, because establishing feedback controls for delegation is part of the authority relationship framework.

The goal of organizing is the coordination of activities, and it is with this last step that the framework is fully established. Even though all the five previous steps are satisfactorily completed, if the members' activities are not tied in, the process can still fail. Members need to know to whom they can go for help and relief.

Open communication lines are an essential part of coordination. The members must be able to communicate freely with one another and with the nurse-leader. Members must know that their authority comes from the nurse-leader. When the nurse-leader is absent, e.g., at a coffee break, she should appoint a substitute to cover her responsibilities while she is gone, and tell the members who the substitute is.

Group members must also know to whom they can turn for assistance. The nurse-leader can arrange this in a flexible way, or she can have a more formal plan. A flexible approach would be when the nurse-leader tells her group members to "help each other" or to go to her when they need her. A more formal arrangement would involve the nurse-leader telling a member to specifically come to her for help, or making it part of one member's assignment to assist another member.

Group members should know when the nurse-leader or other members will be temporarily absent from the units, as in the case of meals or coffee breaks. Again, a formal or informal plan may be established to determine which member will take care of another member's responsibilities while she is away. This is an important organizational function, since it ensures that patients' needs will be met.

Group members, as well as the nurse-leader, must be aware of who is fulfilling which tasks, so that they will be able to find one another when necessary. Posting a list of all the assignments in a central location is a very helpful way of keeping members informed.

Part of coordination involves the nurse-leader having an alternate plan so that, if there are changes or emergencies, the group can continue to function effectively. For example, if one nurse becomes ill and must go home, the nurse-leader must be able to quickly reassign her work to other group members.

The coordination function is extremely important in the process of organizing because it is what brings the whole process together. The six-step process can be employed by all nurse-leaders in any setting, and its use will aid in effective leadership.

AN EXAMPLE OF THE PROCESS OF ORGANIZING IN A NURSING SITUATION

Kathy, a nurse-leader who is a registered nurse in a community hospital, is assigned to be the team leader on the day shift (7 a.m. to 3:30 p.m.) for a group of ten patients on a pediatric unit. The patients are

Susan, an 11-year-old girl who had an appendectomy at 7:00 p.m. the night before. She has never before been hospitalized.

Tony, a 4-year-old boy who has a fractured right femur and has been in traction for 2 weeks.

Peter, a 5-year-old boy who is scheduled for a tonsillectomy and adenoidectomy at 10 a.m. His parents are with him.

Patrick, a 14-month-old boy who has croup and is in a mist tent. It is his third day in the hospital.

Tonya, a 9-year-old girl who fell off her bicycle and sustained a concussion. She will be going home today.

Melissa, a 6-year-old girl who has cerebral palsy. She had a bilateral heel cord lengthening done 2 days ago, and is in casts. She is not retarded.

Russell, a 14-year-old boy who has cystic fibrosis. This is his fourth hospitalization this year, and he is critically ill.

Laura, a 6-month-old baby girl hospitalized because of failure to thrive. She weighed 7 pounds at birth and now weighs 10 pounds. She has gained 3 ounces since yesterday.

Shane, a 2-year-old boy who has diarrhea due to *Salmonella.*

Stephanie, a 16-year-old girl who has anorexia nervosa.

Susan, Patrick, Russell, Laura, Shane, and Stephanie are all in private rooms. Tony and Peter share a room, and so do Tonya and Melissa.

The team members with whom Kathy will work are Jean, a licensed practical nurse (LPN) who has worked on the unit for 2 years and who is very capable, and Paul, a nursing assistant (NA) who has worked on the unit for almost a year. Paul prefers taking care of younger children.

Kathy knows what she has to do. She must proceed with the process of organizing.

Establish Objectives

Kathy's overall goals are: (1) to give all the patients safe, holistic nursing care, and (2) to have all the children and/or their parents indicate, in some way, that they are satisfied with their care. Kathy knows that the first of these objectives is for her team members, and the second for her client group. She is also aware that these objectives fit in with the overall hospital goal, "to provide holistic care for all persons, without regard to age, race, religion, creed, color, sex, or life-style."

Formulate Derivative Objectives

Kathy first prepares specific objectives for each of her clients and team members as follows:

Susan will walk to the playroom and back to her room; she will tell nurses when she has pain.

Tony will play with his punching bag.

Peter will use the puppets to say what is going to happen to him in surgery.

Patrick will be able to eat without coughing.

Tonya and her parents will know what neurological signs they should observe, and will come back to the emergency room if any occur.

Melissa will play in the playroom most of the day.

Russell and his parents will discuss with each other that it is okay for him to die.

Laura will take her feedings without vomiting.

Shane will have only two bowel movements.

Stephanie will eat at least half of the food on her tray and not vomit it.
Jean will give complete care to her assigned patients.
Paul will state that he learned something today.

Kathy remembers several policies and rules that will affect her organizing: parents may visit their children at any time, but other visitors may only visit from 11 a.m. to 1 p.m. and 3 p.m. to 8 p.m.; the pediatrics unit has quiet time from 1 p.m. to 2 p.m., during which all children must be in their rooms and either remain quiet or sleep; all patients going to surgery must be identified by a registered nurse; a hospital staff person or volunteer must accompany to the door every patient who is discharged; licensed practical nurses may not give medications intravenously; respiratory therapists do all respiratory treatments in the hospital. Kathy also knows that a playroom supervisor will be on the unit from 9 a.m. to 1 p.m.

Identify and Classify Activities

Next, Kathy identifies all the activities in the care of each child for the entire shift. When she has set priorities for the activities, her list may look like this:[1]

Susan: turn, cough, and deep breathe; check dressing; pain medications; intake and output; assist with ambulation; a.m. care; make bed.

Tony: assist with eating; skin care; a.m. care; check circulation in foot; check traction; needs to release his energy (punching bag); needs company; make bed.

Peter: preoperative support and puppet play; a.m. care; preoperative medication at 9 a.m.; identify for surgery; tell parents where to wait; make postoperative bed; postoperative checks.

Patrick: check tent; assist with feeding; medications at 9 a.m. and 1 p.m.; intake and output; a.m. care; check diapers; isolation; needs company; make crib.

Tonya: teaching about neurological signs; a.m. care; discharge.

Melissa: check circulation in feet; check casts; a.m. care; to playroom in wheelchair; make bed.

Russell: chest physio; maintain intravenous; medications at 8, 9, and 10 a.m., and noon, and 1 and 3 p.m.; intake and output; emotional support for child and parents; a.m. care; make bed.

Laura: feeding; intake and output; check diapers; a.m. care; sensory and motor stimulation activity; teach parents; make crib.

Shane: check diapers; obtain stool specimen; isolation; maintain intravenous; assist with feeding; a.m. care; play; make crib.

Stephanie: support at meals; calorie count; a.m. care; counseling; schoolwork; diversion; make bed.

Kathy also identifies the unit activities during the shift and ranks them as follows:

8 a.m.: pass breakfast trays—high priority
12 noon: pass lunch trays—high priority
10 a.m. and 2 p.m.: pass fresh water—low priority

---

[1] The authors present this case as an example only. Other nurse-leaders may set other priorities, or make the assignments differently because of their situation.

1 to 2 p.m.: quiet time—high priority
1:30 p.m.: team conference—high priority
3 p.m.: check narcotics—high priority
3:05 p.m.: give report—high priority
Every hour: check orders—high priority

Kathy sees that it will be a very busy day. She knows that Russell is the sickest patient, but Patrick and Laura are both at very high risk; these three are therefore given the highest priority. When Kathy considers her framework for priority setting, she realizes that Russell has obvious needs at all levels. Patrick and Laura have mostly physiological and energy needs.

Kathy also gives Tonya a high priority, so that she can be discharged. Susan, Shane, and Stephanie are given moderate priority because they have mostly safety or structural integrity needs. Tony and Melissa have safety and higher-level needs, so Kathy gives them a low priority.

Peter has some higher-level needs now, which makes him a moderate priority, but he will become a higher priority after surgery because his physiological needs will then be more important. Kathy knows that Peter will probably return to the unit shortly after 11 a.m.

Group Activities

Kathy has already begun to group activities by their priority. Because she has worked with them before, she knows that her team members are used to working within the limits of their job descriptions, with which she is familiar.

Kathy also knows that there are other people she can count on. The playroom supervisor is helpful and dependable. The respiratory therapist has an excellent relationship with Russell. Kathy knows that her head nurse will be supervising the unit, and since they have a very good relationship, Kathy can call on her if she needs help.

Kathy evaluates the material resources that her group will need, and decides that nothing unusual is required. She is sure that all routine supplies will be available, since the ward clerk checks every day and is careful to replenish supplies when necessary.

Kathy groups the following activities for Jean, the LPN:

Laura, Patrick, and Stephanie: pass trays, attend team conference, and check narcotics with a nurse on the next shift. Kathy knows that Laura will take a great deal of time, and that Patrick will need close observation. She thinks Jean will be able to manage this assignment and give the patients complete care.

The assignment Kathy makes for Paul, the NA, includes:

Susan, Shane, Melissa, Tony, and Peter after surgery: pass trays, pass water, and attend team conference. These patients have mostly low-level needs and are young children, so she thinks that Paul will be satisfied. Peter will have higher-level needs after surgery, but Paul has done well with this type of patient before. Moreover, Peter is in the same room with Tony, so Kathy feels that, with her supervision, the assignment will be adequate and Paul will learn something.

Kathy assigns to herself:

Tonya, Russell, and Peter before surgery: check orders, pass trays, lead team conference, and give report. She does not want to be too tied down with patient care, since she needs time to supervise the overall group activity. She also knows that Russel has several intravenous medications, and no one else can do them but her. Although Russell is very ill, he will not need her constantly.

Delegation

Kathy meets with her team to give them their assignments. She asks them if the assignments are agreeable with them, or if they should be modified. Once the assignments are agreed on, she gives both team members a report on their patients and tells them what she expects.

She lets Jean determine how she will carry out her own plan, but makes sure that Jean knows that she should report immediately to Kathy about anything unusual or anything with which she needs help.

Kathy gives Paul a little more direction by suggesting that he may want to check on Susan and Shane first, then give baths to Tony and Melissa. He can then have the playroom supervisor work with Tony and Melissa while he helps Susan and Shane with their care.

Kathy also informs Paul that she herself will take care of Peter until after surgery, but that Paul should make his bed sometime between 10 and 11 a.m. Kathy will let Paul know when she has checked Peter back into the unit, so that he can then take over.

Kathy makes sure that Paul will come to her with any problems or needs. She reminds Jean and Paul that they will have a team conference at 1:30 p.m. about Russell.

Tie Together

Finally, Kathy checks with Jean and Paul about break and lunch times, so that each can cover the other's responsibilities. She tells them when she will be gone, and that the head nurse will cover for her while she is gone.

Kathy makes sure that she has the whole shift organized before beginning her own assignment. She posts the assignments for the head nurse, the ward clerk, and her group to see.

Kathy has left room in her organizational plan for changes. She has kept her own assignment small, so that she can be flexible and ready for any new assignment, such as an admission after Tonya leaves.

Kathy is pleased that she is able to organize effectively. She knows that she will be able to fulfill her responsibility as team leader, because she has reasonable goals and a plan of action to achieve them.

REFERENCES

Beyers, M., & Phillips, C. *Nursing management for patient care.* Boston: Little, Brown, 1979.

Bower, F. L. Nurse as planner. In F. L. Bower and E. O. Bevis (Eds.), *Fundamentals of nursing practice—concepts, roles and functions.* St. Louis: Mosby, 1979.

Jucius, M. J., Deitzer, B. A., & Schlender, W. E. *Elements of managerial action.* Homewood, Ill.: Irwin, 1973.

Koontz, H., & O'Donnell, C. *Management: A systems and contingency analysis of managerial functions.* New York: McGraw-Hill, 1976.

Kron, T. *The management of patient care.* Philadelphia: Saunders, 1976.

Levine, M. E. The four conservation principles of nursing. *Nursing Forum*, 1967, *6*(1), 45–59.

Mager, R. F. *Preparing instructional objectives.* Belmont, Calif.: Fearon, 1962.

Maslow, A. H. *Motivation and personality.* New York: Harper, 1954.

Volante, E. M. Mastering the managerial skill of delegation. *Journal of Nursing Administration*, 1974, *4*(1), 20–22.

Yura, H., & Walsh, M. B. *The nursing process.* New York: Appleton-Century-Crofts, 1978.

ADDITIONAL READINGS

McConnell, E. A. Delegation—myth or reality? *Supervisor Nurse*, 1979, *10*(10), 20–21.

McConnell, E. A. What kind of delegator are you? *Nursing '78*, 1978, *8*(10), 105–110.

Price, M., Franck, P., & Veith, S. *Nursing management: A programmed text.* New York: Springer, 1974.

Wiley, L. The ABCs of time management. *Nursing '78*, 1978, *8*(9), 105–112.

The Nurse-Leader
and the Teaching-Learning
Process

The teaching-learning process is an integral part of the nursing process. Within the nursing process the nurse-leader implements teaching strategies to maximize the learner's health potential. To achieve this potential, learners must learn certain behaviors and skills that will promote, maintain, and restore their health or will allow others to assist them in doing so. The nurse-leader is also in a position to help other members of the interdisciplinary health team assist patients in their quest for health.

LEARNING THEORY

The teaching-learning process in nursing has developed from three views of the learning process: stimulus-response, cognitive-field, and humanistic. Because the definition of learning differs in each of these three families of theories, the definition of teaching also differs. Before defining the teaching-learning process in nursing these three views will be explored briefly.

Stimulus-Response Theory

Learning is a change in behavior or performance. It is a new response brought about by certain conditions, such as need arousal, repeated practice, and reinforcement. Learning occurs when an unmet need produces the motivation to satisfy that need. An unmet need causes tension; the learner desires release from tension and this causes action. The action is the response evoked by teacher-supplied stimuli. Through conditioning— the provision of rewards for the desired response—the learner's needs are met and tension is decreased. Need fulfillment and the accompanying decrease in tension are also rewarding. If this pattern continues, through repeated practice, a habit will form.

Teaching, then, is simply the arrangement of the contingencies of reinforcement (Skinner, 1968, p. 5). The learner is acted upon by the teacher, who controls the learning experience. The teacher specifies the desired response, and the learner, through trial and error, attempts to give the desired response. The learner is rewarded for correct or nearly correct responses.

Cognitive-Field Theory

Learning is an interaction between the learner and the environment that is mediated by the teacher. Learning is internal; within the learner a new insight or cognitive structure is formed or an existing one is altered (Bigge, 1971, p. 199). Understanding is the focus of learning. Because thinking and conceptualizing are the learner's major activities, cognitive development is evaluated by the teacher.

Teaching involves creating situations that make meaningful learning experiences most likely for an individual learner (Cantor, 1953, p. 79). Teaching focuses on the relationships and organization of facts. Learners develop a coding system in their mind to store information. Properly organized subject matter, presented to learners whose cognitive development and processes are correctly understood by the teacher, produces learning (Gage, 1963, p. 138).

Humanistic Theory

Learning is the process of developing one's full potential. Learning can be practicing to make a new skill a habit or incorporating a new idea into one's own understanding, as long as the learner is actively involved in the process and not merely acted upon by the teacher (Gregory, 1917, p. 2). Among the elements involved in this "significant" or "experiential" learning are: (1) the whole person is involved; (2) it is learner-initiated; (3) it is pervasive; (4) it is learner-evaluated; and (5) its essence is meaning (Rogers, 1969, p. 5).

Teaching is the communicating of experience to make learning easier for the learner (Rogers, 1969, p. 105). The learner as a person, not the subject matter, is the focus of teaching and learning. Further, the learner is viewed as the one responsible for the learning. The teacher is available to assist the learner but is not necessarily the initiator of the process.

TEACHING-LEARNING IN NURSING

The nurse-leader teacher utilizes concepts from all three theories to actualize the teaching-learning process in her own unique way. In nursing, teaching-learning is an interactional process in which teacher and learner have specific roles and responsibilities. Through active involvement in the process, learners develop new skills and insights which help them develop their potential as human beings and maximize their health. The teacher also gains skill and insight, particularly in empathy, by relating to each learner as a unique individual.

When teaching a skill such as self-administration of medication, the nurse-leader teacher utilizes the stimulus-response concepts of motivation, repeated practice, and reinforcement. When teaching understanding of diets or medications, the nurse-leader teacher utilizes cognitive-field organization of facts and relationships. She also considers the developmental level of the learner to determine appropriate content and depth.

In every type of teaching-learning experience the nurse-leader teacher utilizes humanistic theory as her framework. Each potential learner, whether patient or interdisciplinary health team member, is considered a unique person in the process of becoming. The teaching-learning process, an integral part of the nursing process, also follows the same steps as the nursing process, i.e., assessing, planning, implementing, and evaluating.

Assessing

Identifying a Need Before teaching or learning can begin, a learning need must be identified. This may be done in several ways. Nurse-leader teachers often *predict* patient learning needs based on nursing knowledge and experience. For instance, a patient requiring bed rest may need some form of active range-of-motion exercises in order to maintain muscle tone. The nurse-leader teacher identifies this patient's need to know how to perform active range-of-motion exercises.

Learning needs are also identified by *interviewing* the potential learner (patient) and finding out about his or her life-style and goals. If a patient enters a health care facility due to illness, the nurse-leader teacher interviews the patient to determine how the illness is perceived and what treatment is expected. By interviewing and listening to the patient, the nurse-leader teacher identifies misconceptions or the need for further information to increase the patient's self-awareness and understanding of the diagnosis.

Nurse-leader teachers observe patients in a variety of settings such as home, work, and school, as well as in health care facilities. *Observation* is another method of identifying learning needs.

While observing a school-aged boy, the nurse-leader teacher notices the child's seeming unfamiliarity with a toothbrush. Through further observation, she may note that the child does not correctly manipulate the toothbrush to ensure adequate dental hygiene. The nurse-leader has identified a potential learning need for this child—to learn to brush his teeth.

Validating the Need Whenever a need is identified by the nurse-leader teacher, it must be validated with the learner. The patient on bed rest may have experienced frequent hospitalizations and be well versed in range-of-motion exercises. However, when the diagnosis is discussed, he or she may omit this information for the sake of brevity. The nurse-leader teacher interviewing this patient must clarify just what the patient knows, so that she does not mistake the omission for a lack of information.

There are several ways to clarify (de Tornyay, 1971, p. 32). One way is simply to ask more questions or make statements that encourage the learner to explain what is meant. "Would you explain that further?" or "I'm not sure what you mean by 'bad blood'" are examples.

Another method of clarifying is to have the learner justify what he or she has said. "What makes you think that your symptoms are due to the medication?" is a question that will show how well the patient has understood.

Prompting the learner may also clarify. Saying to the patient, "You said that you have never been away from your husband before. Is that what is bothering you most?" may allow her to state her true feelings.

The nurse-leader teacher who observed the boy attempting to brush his teeth may have found a child who does not know how to brush his teeth, or she may have found a child who enjoys her attention and is not performing at his usual level. Through repeated observations, she will be able to validate the presence of a real learning need. Clarifying and repeated observations are effective means of validating learning needs with the learner.

The nurse-leader teacher considers additional assessment factors before setting up a teaching plan. These factors are the learner's readiness and motivation.

Readiness Readiness has been defined as the sum of all prior genic effects, all prior incidental experience, and all prior learning, as well as the interaction among these variables (Ausubel, 1963, p. 111). Readiness includes the learner's developmental level, socioeconomic and cultural background, past experiences, and perception of his or her need to learn.

Readiness for any new learning includes the physiological and psychological maturity of the learner. A child cannot be toilet-trained until he or she has sufficient motor control of the bladder and recognizes that micturition is imminent. The child must also be sufficiently psychologically mature to want to please others. Maturity or developmental level is culturally determined. A mature person is one who is capable of fine discriminations, as well as refined and controlled responses to the environment (McDonald, 1959, p. 40).

Readiness is associated with the learner's socioeconomic and cultural background.

A middle-aged man who holds the traditional view that cooking is his wife's job may not feel any need to learn about his diet. If his wife shares this view, she may be very interested in learning about her husband's diet. In this case, the wife is ready for the new learning; her husband is not, and it may therefore be appropriate to teach the wife. However, if the patient travels or frequently eats in restaurants, the nurse-leader teacher must use this data from the patient's life circumstances to increase his readiness. Once he admits that his wife will not always be with him to plan his menus, his need to know about his diet and his readiness will increase.

Readiness also implies the mastery of prerequisites providing a fair chance for success in learning. Prerequisite knowledge for a patient often comes from past experiences rather than formal education. A newly diagnosed juvenile diabetic may have difficulty understanding the relationship of diet, exercise, and insulin management, if she does not understand how her body uses food for energy. If she has a diabetic parent, she may have observed habits in that parent which will make her own learning less difficult.

A sense of importance or relevance of the new learning to the learner's daily life is also a part of readiness. A new student or employee in a hospital may be eager to learn the location and hours of business of the hospital cafeteria in order to meet the need for food.

The physiological and psychological well-being of the learner must be taken into account, because this influences his or her perception of the need to know. Nurse-leader teachers are frequently involved with learners who have health problems. Pain and fatigue may inhibit learning. Denial of the need to know also inhibits learning.

To determine the time when a learner with a health problem is most likely to be ready to learn, the nurse-leader teacher must consider the interaction of the physiological dimensions within the patient. When a patient first becomes ill, he may not recognize that he is ill. After his condition begins to stabilize, his perception of how sick he was is great and, in fact, "feeling sick" predisposes the patient to desire a means of "feeling better" or returning to his usual level of health (Busch & Gallo, 1973, p. 13). Figure 7-1 illustrates the point at which readiness for learning occurs. The psychological lag accounts for the patient's increased complaints after objective evidence indicates that he is recovering and returning to his usual level of health.

Motivation Finally, the nurse-leader teacher must assess the learner's motivation, i.e., willingness to learn. If a learner has identified the need to learn, he or she is more likely to be motivated to achieve this goal.

Since admission, a young woman who has fractures of the left tibia and fibula has been looking forward to going home. One morning she announces to the nurse-leader teacher that she cannot go home until she learns to climb stairs with crutches. This young woman has identified her own learning need and may be considered motivated as well as ready to learn.

Figure 7-1 Time of greatest readiness to learn for clients having a health problem. X = readiness to learn. [*Adapted from C. Hudak, B. Gallo, & T. Lohr (Eds.). Critical care nursing. © 1973 by Lippincott. Used by permission.*]

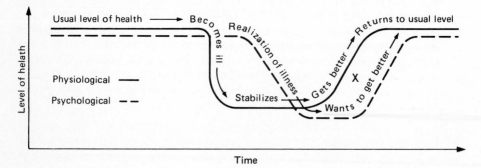

Motivation may be intrinsic or extrinsic. Intrinsic motivation occurs when the learner wants to learn for the sake of learning. Extrinsic motivation occurs when the learner wants to learn for reasons other than the learning (Bigge, 1971, p. 280).

A young boy who tries to play the piano to please his parents exhibits extrinsic motivation. He may practice and attempt to perform well to avoid punishment or to attain praise. He may, however, decide to practice because he finds he enjoys the music and the playing. If he obtains pleasure from the playing, his motivation may change from extrinsic to intrinsic. He will then play because he wants to play and not because of his parents.

Extrinsic motivation is developed through the use of incentives. An incentive is an external influence that causes a learner to act. Depending on the needs of the learner, incentives may be almost anything, e.g., rewards, punishment, or simple explanations. Incentives provided by a significant other may become "double incentives."

Both success and failure may be incentives. If a new female paraplegic is able to take one step using braces and crutches, this may motivate her to try harder to take more steps. Success in taking one step tells her that she is moving toward her goal of walking. When an adolescent fails a driving test and is denied a license, the failure usually encourages him to practice driving so that he can retake the test. Here, failure is the motivation for further learning. However, learning motivated by success is preferable to learning motivated by failure.

Both intrinsic and extrinsic motivation are within the learner. It is *only* the learner who can provide motivation. Often nurse-leader teachers are concerned with "motivating" a patient to learn. This is a misconception. All the nurse-leader teacher can do is to provide incentives to help the patient become extrinsically motivated.

Planning

Setting Goals Once a learning need has been identified and validated with the learner, and the nurse-leader teacher has assessed the learner's readiness and motivation, goals may be determined. The participation of the learner in goal-setting provides the nurse-leader teacher with further data about the learner, the learner's perception of the learning task, and his or her reason for desiring specific information or skills.

An overall goal for the patient on bed rest might be: "maintain muscle tone." Since muscle tone can be maintained in a variety of ways, a more specific objective is needed to provide direction for both teacher and learner. The specific objective might be: "perform active range-of-joint-motion exercises three times each day."

The objective should specify what the patient is to do, and it is helpful if it includes criteria that can be objectively measured. For example, the number of times a performance is expected can easily be counted. Or, a phrase such as "without assistance" can be added to "increase ambulation" to specify walking under one's own power. Objectives may also include criteria that only the patient can evaluate, such as "without developing chest pain." Examples are presented in Table 7-1.

Once the specific objectives are determined from the overall goals, the nurse-

Table 7-1 Setting Learning Objectives from Overall Goals

Overall goal	Specific objective
1 Prevent fatigue	Rest in bed 10 minutes every hour
2 Improve intake	Drink 3000 mL fluid every day
3 Increase ambulation	Walk 50 ft without assistance three times today

leader teacher may proceed with planning the actual teaching-learning experience. The nurse-leader teacher must consider the learner(s), the content to be taught, and the setting, when planning teaching-learning experiences (Chater, 1975).

Learner After the learner's needs, goals, readiness, and motivation have been considered, it is necessary to determine whether there will be one or more learners. When she handles more than one learner, the nurse-leader teacher must find out how much the learners have in common. A group of learners may include patients and their significant others, patients only, or significant others only. The learners may not even be acquainted, and they may have very different backgrounds. The nurse-leader teacher must decide on the size and composition of the group; however, learners must be free to choose whether they wish to be in the group.

Content A primary concern when planning for the content is the nurse-leader teacher's comfort with the subject matter. She must be knowledgeable and have a variety of resources concerning the topic available to her.

The nurse-leader teacher must consider the content so that it can be presented in the best possible way, and select the teaching strategies and methods she will use. She must also consider the amount of time it will take for the material to be taught and learned, and plan the number of sessions and the length of time for each session. She must plan to develop the content, making it relevant to the learners and progressing from what they already know to the new content.

Setting Careful consideration should be given to the setting where teaching-learning experiences are to occur. The number of learners involved affects the choice of setting. There should be a sufficient number of comfortable chairs and tables as well as adequate lighting and ventilation.

Some patients can be taught in their rooms, but a patient who is in a semiprivate room or ward should generally be taken to a private room. A patient who is learning to manage a new colostomy, for example, does not want to be taught in front of roommates.

The setting should have all the necessary equipment and supplies. Defective or inadequate equipment can distract the learner and decrease learning. Therefore, the nurse-leader teacher should test equipment and learn to handle minor repairs such as changing light bulbs in a slide or film projector. If the learner will be practicing deep breathing with an incentive spirometer, supplies must be available and prepared prior to the teaching-learning experience, so that time is not wasted.

The location of the classroom is important. Patients must be able to get to it easily either by themselves or with assistance. The nurse-leader teacher can either give the patient directions or arrange to have the patient brought to the classroom.

Teaching should be scheduled at a time that is convenient for the patient, who should not have to worry about missing treatments or tests as a result of attending a class. Teaching should also be scheduled at a time when the patient is awake and alert. If an elderly man is accustomed to napping after his noon meal, it would be unwise to schedule him for a 1 p.m. session.

Implementing

Teaching Strategies Once the planning has been completed, the actual teaching can begin. The nurse-leader teacher can use a variety of strategies in her teaching. Strategies are techniques the teacher uses to foster learning.

Setting the Stage Creating a comfortable atmosphere in which learning can occur, or setting the stage, is the first strategy. The nurse-leader teacher should be friendly, warm, and kind to the learners, calling them by name and maintaining good eye contact.

There are many barriers which the nurse-leader teacher can remove so that learning can be facilitated. Two such barriers are fear of the unknown and preconceptions about the presumed known. If a positive first impression is created, fear and misconceptions will be diminished, and learning will occur more easily. During the first meeting, the nurse-leader teacher can provide a framework that clearly tells the learner what he or she can expect. Objectives are reviewed and agreed upon, and the relationship of past learning or experience to the present learning task is made explicit.

Giving learners an overall view of the learning they will experience is helpful in the beginning. The overview can be accomplished by listing or outlining the entire course of study or practice, then specifying the time frame within which it will occur. Learners then know what the end point or destination is, as well as how they are going to get there.

Providing the learner with adequate expectations will also decrease fear and remove barriers to learning. If a learner is expected to repeat a performance after a demonstration is given, he or she should be informed of this. If the learner knows that the nurse-leader teacher will perform the task before the learner is asked to do so, this will help alleviate anxiety. Often, the consequences of an action create fear. Allowing a learner to inject water into an orange before injecting insulin into himself is a reassuring experience.

Varying Stimuli Even if a teacher is a very interesting lecturer, both she and her learners would quickly become bored if that were the only method she used. Some repetition is helpful, but too much dulls the response of the learner and leads to boredom. To avoid monotony, the teacher will vary the stimuli, or input, the learner encounters.

It is generally thought that any change or deviation from a standard will result in a higher attention span and thus enhance learning. Varying the stimuli increases learners' interest and serves as an aid to memory.

There are numerous ways to vary the stimuli. One is simply by using the voice. Learners quickly get bored if their teacher speaks in the same tone, especially if the tone is quiet and soothing. The nurse-leader teacher can vary her voice quality by speaking loudly, softly, quickly, or slowly, as is appropriate to the subject.

Using planned periods of silence promotes thinking on the part of the learner. Too much silence, or long periods of silence, may cause anxiety because the learner does not know what is coming next. Silence can convey acceptance, disagreement, sharing, or ignoring.

Just as the voice can demonstrate enthusiasm, so can gestures. Hand, arm, and head gestures are most commonly used. Too much shaking of hands or banging of fists may become repetitive and thus boring or distracting. Helpful gestures are ones that emphasize the important or major points.

Complete body movement is also a gesture. Walking to the blackboard and writing on it varies the stimuli. It also focuses the learner's attention on what is being written. Merely standing at the blackboard (or overhead projector) and writing can again become monotonous.

Audiovisual materials can add variety to the teaching-learning experience. Many drug and medical product companies provide pamphlets, flip charts, and slide and tape series about diagnoses and medications, which the learner can use in conjunction with regular meetings with the nurse-leader teacher.

The teacher might show films, play records, or invite guest speakers to vary the classroom experience. The classroom furniture might be rearranged, or posters could be placed around the room. Assignments can also be varied so that the routine does not become monotonous. A diabetic patient attending a series of classes on treatments for diabetes will quickly tire of an assignment to read one pamphlet before every class.

It must be remembered, however, that too much variation is as bad as too little. The stimuli chosen must be appropriate to the learner, the content, and the setting.

Using Examples and Models The use of examples and models is another way of varying the stimuli, and a useful strategy in the teaching-learning experience. An example is an item or illustration that represents something else. A model is a miniature or replica of something.

Examples must be chosen carefully. Examples are meant to enhance or demonstrate a concept; they may, however, represent more than one idea, some of which may be inappropriate. If a patient is taught that a cannula is like a canal, the patient may not remember the word "cannula" because the word "canal" is so similar.

Examples should be appropriate, clear, and relevant. The concept should not get lost in the example, or it will be the example that is remembered and not the concept. This may happen when the teacher least expects it. For example, a mother might have explained to her 6-year-old daughter that the child's dead grandmother just "slept away." The mother's intention was to convey to her daughter that death is not painful. However, the child becomes afraid to go to sleep at night because she now associates sleep with death.

Models are helpful in many situations, particularly when teaching patients about anatomy and physiology. Being able to hold a plastic heart in one's hand and take it apart to see how it works is better than just hearing about a heart or even seeing a picture.

Like examples, models should be appropriate, clear, and relevant. It is not necessary to show a patient a whole skeleton to illustrate a fractured hand. Also, the size difference between the model and the real thing must be remembered and explained to the learner. The patient examining a model of a heart will not know whether the model is the same size as a human heart, larger, or smaller.

Sometimes models can be the "real thing." There is no better way to teach an elderly woman about her total hip surgery than to show her a total hip prosthesis. Other prostheses can be used in the same way, e.g., mitral valves or silicone implants for augmentation mammoplasties and other joints to be replaced. However, such prostheses are expensive and may not be available in every setting.

One of the oldest recognized beliefs about learning is the *law of the lesson*, which states that, when teaching a new subject, it must somehow be related to the known and the familiar (Gregory, 1917, p. 58). To do this, simple or known examples should be presented first, then more complex examples can follow. If a 50-year-old woman has a radical mastectomy, Betty Ford or Happy Rockefeller could be used as simple examples—the known for her. The patient herself is the more complex example, the unknown.

Questioning Questioning is another method of varying the stimuli in a teaching-learning experience, but it is also an important teaching strategy in itself. There are two types of questions: (1) questions that seek answers and (2) rhetorical questions, or questions asked simply for effect that do not require answers. The nurse-leader teacher will want to use both types.

Questions that seek answers are of three kinds: factual or descriptive, clarifying, and higher-order (deTornyay, 1971, p. 31). Factual or descriptive questions are the most frequently asked questions; they do not, however, promote the greatest depth of learning. They do help learners memorize, since factual questions seek a simple answer. Clarifying questions are more demanding than factual questions because they urge learners to give more than a superficial response (deTornyay, 1971, p. 32). Higher-order questions demand most from the learner. Higher-order questions force learners to solve problems and think abstractly (deTornyay, 1971, p. 36). They promote learning of the greatest depth.

Ordinarily, the nurse-leader teacher asks questions in the order of factual, clarifying, and higher-order, because this is another way of moving from the known to the unknown. The following example demonstrates the use of asking questions of increasing complexity.

Teacher: What substance is secreted from the beta cells of the islets of Langerhans in the pancreas? (factual)
Learner: Insulin.
Teacher: Why is it secreted? (descriptive)
Learner: To remove the sugar from the blood.

Teacher: How does that happen? (clarifying)
Learner: Sugar is in food, but it can't be used unless insulin joins with it and helps it get into the cells.
Teacher: Right. Now what implications are there for a person whose pancreas does not secrete insulin? (higher-order)

It is possible to begin with a clarifying question such as, "How does sexual intercourse affect the heart?" Then, if the learner cannot answer, the teacher can go back and ask factual questions which will help the learner answer the clarifying question by putting facts together.

The higher-order question may be asked initially as a rhetorical question. The learner is stimulated to think and focus on the concept. After some information is presented, the question may be asked again, this time seeking an answer. Rhetorical questions help learners to focus on the content and may encourage them to ask questions. Rhetorical questions may be the only questions used in a lecture for a large group.

Certain principles must be remembered when asking questions. The first and most important is to ask only *one* question at a time. Learners must be allowed to answer, or think about an answer, before the next question is asked, or they will be unable to learn.

In addition, the question itself must have a single focus and not ask more than one question within itself. Asking a nursing mother, "Is there a relationship between your diet and your baby's bowel movements, and what is it?" is not only confusing to the mother, it also assumes the answer.

Questions should also be free from bias. "You want to learn about your emphysema, don't you?" implies that the person has no choice and will be taught, regardless of his or her feelings.

Giving Feedback   Giving feedback is not just a teaching strategy, it is an indispensable part of learning. Studies have shown that knowing one has made progress is essential for effective learning (Blair, Jones, & Simpson, 1962, p. 182).

Feedback may be positive (reinforcement) or negative (constructive criticism). Positive reinforcement increases the chances that a desired behavior will reoccur. It is therefore given when a desired behavior has occurred. Positive reinforcement may be verbal or nonverbal. The nurse-leader teacher may respond with "yes," "right," "very good," or other similar words. She may also smile, touch the learner, nod her head "yes," or step toward the learner to indicate that the desired behavior was accomplished.

In addition to reinforcement for successful performance, learners need to know about their mistakes (Hilgard, 1956, p. 487) and to have some means of correcting them immediately (Blair et. al., 1962, p. 182). Constructive criticism is a method used to help learners learn from their mistakes. To provide constructive criticism, the teacher must tell learners what they did correctly as well as what they did incorrectly. Then the learner and teacher can work together to find the desired behavior.

Constructive criticism may become a negative reinforcer, i.e., something that decreases the chances that a behavior will be repeated. Negative reinforcers include threats, punishment, and pain. "You will not be able to go home if you don't learn to walk" is a negative reinforcer. However, learning controlled by rewards is usually preferable to learning controlled by punishment (Hilgard, 1956, p. 486).

Silence may be used as feedback and can be positively or negatively reinforcing, depending on the circumstances. The nonverbal behavior of the teacher will usually tell the learner whether the silence is positive or negative. A teacher who is frowning or who appears tense is giving negative reinforcement, while a teacher who is smiling and relaxed is giving positive reinforcement. Sometimes silence is an urging to go on, and this is also positive reinforcement.

For the most effective learning, positive reinforcement must come almost immediately after the desired behavior. In addition, the learner must be able to connect the reinforcer with the behavior he or she has exhibited (Watson, 1964, p. 27). It is not as reinforcing to tell a group of learners that they have all done well as it is to tell each member of the group that he or she did well.

Intermittent reinforcement can be very effective, and is required in many instances. A nurse-leader teacher who is teaching a LaMaze class to eight couples cannot possibly reinforce each couple for each correct action they perform. She can, however, reinforce them intermittently. If the proportion of responses that she reinforces is steadily reduced, the couple's behavior may be maintained with very few reinforcers (Skinner, 1968, p. 159). The couple will have learned to reinforce themselves. It is important for learners to be able to reinforce themselves because a teacher will not always be there to provide reinforcement.

Another reason for using intermittent reinforcement is that too frequent reinforcement can reduce the power of the reinforcer. If a teacher always says, "that's good," those words will soon mean nothing to the learner.

Reviewing the outline of study periodically is a method of intermittent feedback that keeps the learner informed of progress, and reinforces the objectives to be accomplished. The teacher is able to keep the learner motivated by providing feedback and satisfying the learner's needs, which will be met by goal achievement (McDonald, 1959, p. 525).

If sufficient feedback, either positive or negative, is not provided, behavior will become extinct, that is, become weaker or completely disappear. For example, extinction of pain behavior is the principle behind behavior modification therapy in pain management units.

Providing for Retention and Transfer   An important strategy in the teaching-learning process is that of providing for retention and transfer. Since the ultimate goal of the process is to promote desirable changes in performance that will carry into new situations (Blair et. al., 1962, p. 280), the learner must be able to remember and use what has been learned.

Retention means remembering correctly and implies recognition as well as recall (Hulse, Diese, & Egeth, 1975, p. 346). Transfer of learning occurs when learning in one situation influences the learner's performance in another situation (Bigge, 1971, p. 243).

Retention and transfer are not automatic. Techniques the nurse-leader teacher can use to help the learner remember what has been learned and use it in everyday life include identical elements, overlearning, general principles, active involvement and performance feedback.

Retention and transfer are dependent on teaching-learning experiences that use lifelike situations. What is learned is most likely to be available for use if it is learned in a situation similar to the one in which it is to be used (Watson, 1964, p. 31). The number of *identical elements* in both interpersonal and physical characteristics of the setting will maximize retention and transfer. For example, if a diabetic is expected to test his urine at home and at work, a bathroom would normally be a setting with identical elements. But if the diabetic worked at mobile construction sites with no running water in the portable bathroom, he should be taught a urine testing method that is not dependent on water for dilution.

Obviously, the best learning situation for identical elements is the setting in which performance usually occurs. It would be advantageous for the nurse-leader teacher to arrange, when possible, for teaching-learning at home.

Retention and transfer are improved by overlearning. *Overlearning* refers to the continuation of practice or repetition after the desired response has been given. By observing the repeated performance of the correct behavior, the nurse-leader teacher has the opportunity to reinforce the behavior, as well as to make sure the performance is correct each time. High levels of practice and overlearning increase the number of correct responses and help reassure the learner.

A patient with chronic obstructive pulmonary disease (COPD) may need to use a hand-held nebulizer for inhalation therapy at home. By encouraging the patient to assemble, use, and clean the nebulizer himself, the nurse-leader teacher can observe, evaluate, and reinforce this behavior. In addition, she can reassure the patient that he is using the correct procedure, even if sputum production does not occur each time the nebulizer is used.

Material that is meaningful to the learner is retained much better than material that is not. Meaningfulness consists of relationships among facts (Bigge, 1971, p. 289). If the nurse-leader teacher teaches logical reasoning by asking the learner to solve problems, the learner gains experience in reasoning, and learning will be more permanent (Seagoe, 1956, p. 257). Using *general principles* ensures that memory loss will not mean total loss, because what remains permits reconstruction of details (Bruner, 1960, pp. 24–25).

When teaching crutch-walking, the nurse-leader teacher may provide the learner with a general principle such as, "always put your best foot forward." The learner attempting to climb up or down stairs should have little difficulty because of the guiding principle.

Feedback is given in the teaching-learning process to make learners aware of their progress. *Performance feedback* for retention and transfer refers to feedback given in the situation for which the learner was being prepared. For example, a patient might be taught in a clinic how to take his own blood pressure and given feedback for correct performance. To provide for retention and transfer, a public health nurse might later visit the patient at home and find that he is correctly checking his blood pressure. The nurse would then give performance feedback to encourage the patient to continue the behavior.

Often, printed material is available for use by patients. It is important for the nurse-leader teacher to remember that trying to recall what has been read is more conducive to learning than rereading the material (Watson, 1964, p. 30). The nurse-leader teacher would instruct the learner to summarize the material in her own words, and later ask her to reproduce it. The nurse-leader teacher then reinforces the learner's correct summary. The fact that the learner can recall and summarize the information will also provide performance feedback because of the sense of satisfaction that the accomplishment gives.

Research indicates that *active involvement* of the learner greatly increases retention and transfer. Learners remember 90 percent of what they say as they *do* something. The nurse-leader teacher can greatly increase the learners' retention and transfer by having them explain what they are doing while they are doing it. Further, just talking through what has been learned will ensure about 80 percent retention of material. Audiovisual aids help retention by stimulating the senses; the learner, without saying anything, may remember about 50 percent of what has been seen and heard. Unfortunately, hearing or seeing alone provides only 20 to 30 percent retention—a loss of 70 to 80 percent of the learning (Medearis, 1973, p. 320). The nurse-leader teacher will provide for retention and transfer by involving the patient actively in the learning process.

Teaching Methods The nurse-leader teacher must be aware of and use various teaching methods, as well as teaching strategies. Teaching methods are the ways in which the teacher or learner conducts the teaching-learning experience. Teaching methods can be classified as *teacher-centered* or *learner-centered*. Specific teaching methods may be placed on a continuum ranging from wholly teacher-centered methods to wholly learner-centered methods (see Figure 7-2).

Teacher-centered methods tend to be the traditional ways of teaching. Objectives are determined by the teacher and emphasis is usually on cognitive learning. In the teaching-learning experience, interaction is directed toward the teacher. The teacher determines the activities for the learners and keeps them focused on the content (McKeachie, 1963, p. 1134).

Learner-centered methods tend to be more free and open. Objectives are defined by the learners, or by the learners with the teacher. Emphasis may be placed on affective and attitudinal change as well as on cognitive learning. Moreover, there is more interaction in the teaching-learning experience—and as much between learners as between teacher and learner. The learners may decide on their own activities, and sharing of personal experiences is encouraged. A "group feeling" tends to develop among the learners (McKeachie, 1963, p. 1134). Figure 7-3 is an illustration of interaction and communication in teacher-centered and learner-centered teaching methods.

Lecture The oldest and probably most used teaching method is the lecture. In the true lecture, the teacher does all the talking, and rarely, if ever, are audiovisual aids used. Although it is frequently criticized, the lecture method has a number of advan-

Figure 7-2 Continuum of teaching methods.

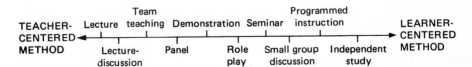

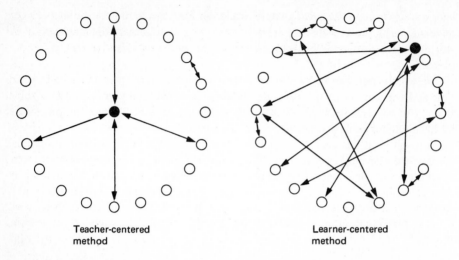

Teacher-centered
method

Learner-centered
method

Figure 7-3 Comparison of interaction in teacher-centered and learner-centered teaching methods.
(● = teacher, ○ = learner.)

tages. It is the best way of transmitting a great deal of well-organized content to a large
group of learners in a short period of time. The lecture can be used to direct learners'
thoughts in a particular direction as it emphasizes or clarifies facts from a book. Further, it is a way of exposing a large number of learners to a recognized authority or
specialist in a field (deTornyay, 1971, p. 66). Learners can also tape-record (with permission) a lecture for their future use.

The lecture has several disadvantages, not the least of which is that most teachers
do not know how to lecture. Lecturing is a skill which must be developed.[1] Learners
may become passive recipients of information during a lecture. If learners are trying to
understand concepts or develop problem-solving skills, they need to be active partici-
pants in the teaching-learning experience to do so effectively.

Because they cannot respond during a lecture, learners may "get lost," i.e., become confused, so that they give up and consequently learn little. Learners may also
become bored and think about unrelated topics or even fall asleep. In addition,
because learners are often trying to take notes rapidly, they forget to, or cannot, think
about what they are hearing, and learning is thus decreased.

There are very few times when a nurse-leader teacher needs to use the lecture
method. It might be used for staff development or for continuing education presenta-
tions to a very large group, or when a specific amount of information must be covered
within a short time span.

Lecture-Discussion The lecture-discussion method is the modern way of lecturing
using audiovisual aids and allowing learner participation through asking and answering
questions. Much discussion and many studies have considered the question of which
method—lecture or discussion—is the better learning method. The lecture-discussion

[1] An excellent discussion of how to prepare and give lectures can be found in K. E. Eble.
The craft of teaching. San Francisco: Jossey-Bass, 1977.

provides the best of both methods, since the teacher can provide sufficient content and still involve the learner. Both teacher and learners can ask questions—to obtain more facts, to clarify, or to stimulate thinking. The teacher is still in control, but maintains contact with the learners.

The limitations to the lecture-discussion method are mainly those of the lecture method. Only a certain number of the learners will become involved; the rest will remain passive or get lost. The lecture-discussion method can be used with a much smaller group of learners than the lecture, but it is not a good method to use with a single learner.

The nurse-leader teacher can use the lecture-discussion method for teaching groups of patients about their diagnoses, medications, or treatments. Much teaching in nursing utilizes the lecture-discussion method.

Team Teaching   Team teaching is a method in which two or more teachers, who have different knowledge and abilities, work together to teach a group of learners. The teaching-learning experience is basically a discussion among the teachers and the learners.

The team-teaching method has advantages for both the learners and the teachers. The learners are exposed to the skills of more than one teacher and, therefore, may learn more. Furthermore, because teachers often have differing opinions, learners realize that there may be more than one correct way of looking at a topic and are forced to consider a variety of solutions, and to form their own opinions.

The teachers also benefit because they can learn from one another. Teachers may learn content as well as teaching skills. Further, they may learn to cooperate and support one another rather than to compete—although competition can occur when teachers teach together.

Team teaching also has disadvantages for both learners and teachers. The greatest disadvantage for the learners is that the teaching-learning experience may become disorganized and confusing if it is not well planned. Bright students usually like the team-teaching method because they get involved, ask questions, and are stimulated to think. Less bright students may have more difficulty because of too much stimulation.

The disadvantage for teachers is the time involved. Team teaching requires much more time than teaching alone, and for that reason it is more costly. Extensive cooperative planning is essential for effective team teaching.

The nurse-leader teacher can utilize the team-teaching method in a number of situations. She may teach groups of patients about discharge planning with an occupational therapist, about diets with a dietitian, or about home care with another nurse-leader teacher.

Panel   A panel presentation is a teaching method in which a small group of teachers sit on a panel in front of a group of learners. A moderator directs the process, in which each teacher presents some portion of a topic; this is followed by a discussion among the presenters on the whole topic. After that, the group of learners may ask questions and interact with members of the panel.

The strength of the panel as a teaching method is that each member of the panel is an expert on the topic and, therefore, learners are exposed to a variety of opinions and concepts. Further, learners participate in the teaching-learning experience by asking questions. They may also be able to identify with members of the panel and can learn more because they do.

A limitation to the panel is that panel members may speak for longer than they were asked, and it is difficult and disruptive for the moderator to interrupt. If the presenters take too much time, what is lost or shortened is the time in which learners may interact with the panel.

An example of a panel could be a nurse, a physician, and a physical therapist teaching a group of parents about cerebral palsy. The nurse-leader teacher could be either a panel member or the moderator. Another panel might include a rehabilitated male quadriplegic and his wife and a rehabilitated female paraplegic and her husband.

Demonstration   The demonstration method is a teaching method that relies heavily on the concept of modeling, or imitation. In the demonstration method, the teacher performs a behavior, and, at the same time, explains to the learners why each step is done. A knowledge of the underlying principles of a procedure is as important as the physical skills involved. As the teacher demonstrates, she encourages learners to ask questions and be involved in the teaching-learning experience.

The next step in the demonstration method is practice by the learners. At this time, learners model themselves after the example of the teacher, i.e., they try to do exactly what she did and remember why she did it. It is important that the teacher supervise the practice, so that she can give feedback, reinforcing the desired behaviors and correcting any undesired behavior. Distributed practice, i.e., short practice periods interspersed with rest or other activities, has been shown to promote greater learning than massed practice, i.e., long, uninterrupted practice periods (Bigge, 1971, p. 186). Therefore, the teacher will schedule brief practice sessions over 1 or more days, so that the greatest learning can occur.

A return demonstration by the learner to the teacher is the final step in the demonstration method. The teacher allows the learner to perform the skill uninterrupted, unless the learner is likely to be injured or to injure another. If errors are made, the learner must practice more and do another return demonstration.

If the teacher is seen by the learner as a friendly and helpful expert, and the learner is reinforced for performing the activity, modeling and learning of the desired behavior will be more successful (Goldstein & Sorcher, 1974, p. 28). Further, teaching which is explicit and detailed; which moves from simple to complex; which is repetitive enough to foster overlearning, but not cause boredom; and which contains little extraneous behavior (behavior that should *not* be modeled) will promote the greatest modeling and learning (Goldstein & Sorcher, 1974, p. 28).

Advantages to the demonstration method include (1) it is probably the best method for teaching skills; (2) it can be used with one or many learners, and (3) learners are encouraged to be involved and are able to apply their skills immediately.

A disadvantage of the demonstration method is the amount of time involved. The teaching demonstration may take three times as long to perform as the actual procedure itself. The time practice takes will depend upon the individual learner, but time must also be set aside for the return demonstration.

The nurse-leader teacher uses the demonstration method a great deal in teaching both patients and staff. It may be used, for example, to demonstrate irrigating a colostomy, bathing a baby, counting a pulse, or changing a dressing.

Role Play Role play is a teaching method in which the teacher identifies a situation and selects learners to play the parts of the persons involved. There is no script; the learner-players interact with one another as if they were the characters. Following the acting, a discussion is held to analyze and synthesize what happened. Role play can be used to develop interpersonal skills and awareness of feelings in learners.

The advantage of role play is that it involves learners in the teaching-learning experience. The problem is that several learners are necessary. Some learners must observe and some must act, so that the group can later discuss the interpretations and feelings of those who observed as well as those who acted out the roles. Moreover, role play is not always successful—learners may feel self-conscious about playing the roles, or they may treat role play as a game instead of a teaching-learning experience.

Role play is used mostly in psychiatric nursing. For example, parents and adolescents may be able to gain insights about their conflicts through role playing. Assertiveness can also be taught with this method.

Seminar The seminar is a teaching method in which a small group of learners (five to twelve) come together to analyze a problem chosen for discussion. Usually, the seminar extends over a period of time. Each learner is responsible for sharing knowledge and interacting with other learners. The main purpose of the seminar is to foster divergent thinking and encourage problem solving.

The teacher functions as a group member and is therefore also a learner. However, in the beginning, learners often expect the teacher to be the leader. The teacher must exhibit the behaviors she expects of the learners so that the learners can assume leadership and management of the seminar.

The most important benefit of the seminar is that learners have been shown to learn better in small groups than in large ones (Schein, 1972, p. 111). Learners are actively involved and must study and prepare in order to participate fully.

The greatest disadvantage of the seminar may be that many types of group discussions are called "seminars" when they are not. The word "seminar" is often used for conferences and workshops in which only lectures occur. Learners who were anticipating a true seminar may be unclear about what is expected of them. Another disadvantage is that, unless learners are prepared, and join in the discussion, little learning will occur.

Due to its nature, the seminar can rarely be used by the nurse-leader teacher. It might be used when a group of nurses or other interdisciplinary health team members meet to discuss a general topic such as "Ethical Issues in the Care of the Dying Patient." The members of the group would pursue the topic over a period of time, and each learner would prepare for each meeting.

Small Group Discussion The small group discussion is a teaching method often used by the nurse-leader teacher. Small group discussions of any kind should not be used to teach new content, but to increase the depth and breadth of knowledge about a topic with which members are already familiar.

The nurse-leader teacher might use this teaching method when she plans a team conference on a topic such as amyotrophic lateral sclerosis. Most, if not all the nurses, will know something about this condition. However, because it is so rare, and because patients with the diagnosis are seldom seen, it is a good subject to review when a patient with the disease is admitted.

The nurse-leader teacher often uses small group discussions to teach patients. Classes about certain diagnoses might be scheduled so that patients may come together to share information, or to learn from each other.

Programmed Instruction   Programmed instruction is a teaching method in which the learner learns a topic by following a program. The content is written in a sequence of steps and questions and answers are provided within the program. The learner reads the material, answers the questions, and is provided with immediate feedback about the answers.

Programmed instruction may be provided by a book or by a teaching machine or computer. The teacher decides what the learner must learn and provides the learner with the programmed instruction. Then it is the learner's responsibility to learn the content of the program.

The major advantage of the programmed instruction is that learners can proceed at their own rate. Also, they can return to review sections with which they had difficulty. In addition, learners can use the program at their own discretion. If the program is a book, learners are also free to choose the learning environment that they prefer.

A disadvantage of programmed instruction is that a learner may answer a question with a correct answer, but one that is different from the given one. The learner may not recognize that both answers are correct.

The nurse-leader teacher can use programmed instruction effectively with patients. Some programmed instruction units may be purchased, or the nurse-leader teacher may prepare her own. Topics might include "How the Heart Works," "Hypertension," or "The Process of Labor."

Independent Study   Independent study is a teaching method in which the learner is given the greatest responsibility for learning. The underlying assumption is that a learner will learn more if allowed to work independently.

In an independent study, one or more learners select a topic, write objectives, and plan to meet and evaluate the objectives. Learners then share this information with a teacher who agrees to help them meet their goals. The teacher plays a greater or lesser part in the teaching-learning experience, depending upon the agreement that is made between teacher and learners.

The premise of the independent study teaching method is that a learner who selects his or her own study will be motivated to complete the project and learn. An advantage for the teacher who has several learners working on independent studies is that he or she is free to assist each one on an individual basis at the time each desires help.

The independent study is not suitable for the learner who has poor study habits and who lacks motivation. Ordinarily, these learners should not attempt independent studies, but occasionally they do. Nor should it be used by teachers who believe that the learner is totally responsible for the learning and, as a result, give little or no guidance to the learner.

The independent study will most likely be used by the nurse-leader herself, as she works to continue her education. It may also be used by the nurse-leader teacher with certain learners. For example, a high school student might wish to study rheumatic fever because her brother had had the disease. The student could work independently, using the school nurse as her teacher.

Other teaching methods exist, as well as variations of the methods described. The nurse-leader teacher will choose the method which best suits her own needs as well as the needs of the learner. She will want to choose a method appropriate for the learner, the content, and the setting. Figure 7-2 illustrates the specific methods which have been described in this section.

Evaluating

It is essential that the teaching-learning process include some means whereby the nurse-leader teacher and the learner can judge whether or not the learner has learned. The evaluation of learning in the teaching-learning process is identical to the evaluation of expected outcomes in the nursing process. The learner's performance is compared with the objectives specified during planning to see if the learner has or has not met the objectives. If the learner has done so, then the identified need should have been met. If not, the teaching-learning process should continue.

If the learner has not learned, that is, not met the objectives, there are several possible explanations. The nurse-leader teacher must review each component of the teaching-learning process to find out why learning has not occurred. The identified need may not have been the real learning need. Perhaps the strategies and methods did not suit the individual learner, or were not appropriate for the content. Often, the learner's levels of readiness and motivation change over time. A reassessment of these areas will provide the nurse-leader teacher with needed information to begin to guide the learner through the teaching-learning process again.

CONCLUSION

The components of the teaching-learning process outlined in this chapter refer to planned teaching that occurs within the nursing process. Teaching and learning also occur in an unplanned or incidental context. Incidental teaching-learning occurs whenever a patient asks the nurse-leader a question and she answers it. This happens on a daily basis as patients inquire about medications, clinic hours, and any number of other health-related matters.

Incidental teaching-learning also occurs more subtly in ways the nurse-leader may not anticipate. Because "nurse" is defined differently by each individual the nurse-leader encounters, she must be aware of the influence of her behavior on the unidentified learner. "Nurse" implies a certain role. A role is a set of expectations about the appropriate behavior of an individual in a given position within a social system (McDonald, 1959, p. 483).

For example, a nurse-leader functioning as a coronary-rehabilitation counselor must encourage her patients who experienced myocardial infarctions (MI) to refrain

Table 7-2   The Teaching-Learning Process in Relation to the Nursing Process

Assessment	Planning	Implementation	Evaluation
Identify need	Specify objectives	Use strategies	Observe learner
Validate need	Consider learner	Use methods	Determine if learner has met objectives
Determine readiness	Consider content		
Determine motivation	Consider setting		
	Select strategies and methods		

from smoking. Although the nurse-leader herself does not have heart disease, her patients will expect that she, too, will not smoke. If the nurse-leader smells of smoke, the MI patient-learner will be less likely to comply with her teaching.

Because the nurse-leader is always being viewed by her patients as "nurse," it is important that she examine her own behavior and attitudes. The nurse-leader will want to portray positive health behavior to her patients. Since incidental teaching-learning occurs so frequently, it is important that the nurse-leader incorporate the components of the teaching-learning process for planned teaching into her moment-to-moment encounters with patients.

The components of the teaching-learning process as they relate to the nursing process are summarized in Table 7-2.

REFERENCES

Ausubel, D. P. *The psychology of meaningful verbal learning.* New York: Grune & Stratton, 1963.

Bigge, M. L. *Learning theories for teachers.* New York: Harper and Row, 1971.

Blair, G. M., Jones, R. S., & Simpson, R. H. *Educational psychology.* New York: Macmillan, 1962.

Bruner, J. S. *The process of education.* Cambridge, Mass.: Harvard University Press, 1960.

Busch, K. D., & Gallo, B. M. Emotional response to illness. In C. M. Hudak, B. M. Gallo, & T. Lohr (Eds.), *Critical care nursing.* Philadelphia: Lippincott, 1973.

Cantor, N. *The teaching←→learning process.* New York: Dryden, 1953.

Chater, S. Conceptual framework for curriculum development. *Nursing Outlook,* 1975, *23,* 428–433.

de Tornyay, R. *Strategies for teaching nursing.* New York: Wiley, 1971.

Gage, N. L. (Ed.). *Handbook of research on teaching.* Chicago: Rand McNally, 1963.

Goldstein, A. P., & Sorcher, M. *Changing supervisor behavior.* New York: Pergamon, 1974.

Gregory, J. M. *The seven laws of teaching.* Chicago: Pilgrim, 1917.

Hilgard, E. R. *Theories of learning.* New York: Appleton-Century-Crofts, 1956.

Hulse, S. H., Deese, J., & Egeth, H. *The psychology of learning.* New York: McGraw-Hill, 1975.

McDonald, F. J. *Educational psychology*. San Francisco: Wadsworth, 1959.

McKeachie, W. J. Research on teaching at the college and university level. In N. L. Gage (Ed.), *Handbook of research on teaching*. Chicago: Rand McNally, 1963.

Medearis, N. D. Planning for the training and development of the critical care nursing staff. In C. M. Hudak, B. M. Gallo, & T. Lohr (Eds.), *Critical care nursing*. Philadelphia: Lippincott, 1973.

Rogers, C. R. *Freedom to learn*. Columbus, Ohio: Merrill, 1969.

Schein, E. H. *Professional education*. New York: McGraw-Hill, 1972.

Seagoe, M. V. *A teacher's guide to the learning process*. Dubuque, Iowa: Brown, 1956.

Skinner, B. F. *The technology of teaching*. New York: Appleton-Century-Crofts, 1968.

Watson, G. What psychology can we trust? In R. E. Ripple (Ed.), *Learning and human abilities: Educational psychology*. New York: Harper & Row, 1964.

ADDITIONAL READINGS

Block, J. H. *Mastery learning*. New York: Holt, Rinehart, & Winston, 1971.

Brown, G. I. *Human teaching for human learning*. New York: Viking, 1971.

Cooper, S. S. Methods of teaching—revisited. *Journal of Continuing Education in Nursing*, 1978, *9*(4), 24–26.

Gagné, R. M. *The conditions of learning*. New York: Holt, Rinehart, & Winston, 1970.

Guinée, K. K. *Teaching and learning in nursing*. New York: Macmillan, 1978.

Pohl, M. L. *The teaching function of the nursing practitioner*. Dubuque, Iowa: Brown, 1978.

Pugh, E. J. Dynamics of teaching-learning interaction. *Nursing Forum*, 1976, *15*, 47–58.

Redman, B. K. *The process of patient teaching in nursing*. St. Louis: Mosby, 1976.

Schweer, J. E., & Gebbie, K. M. *Creative teaching in clinical nursing*. St. Louis: Mosby, 1976.

Sheahan, J. Methods of learning, planning for teaching. *Nursing Times*, 1976, *72*, 1405–1407.

Stevens, B. J. The teaching-learning process. *Nurse Educator*, 1976, *1*(1), 9–20.

Chapter 8

The Nurse-Leader
and the Decision-Making Process

The nurse-leader is constantly involved in the decision-making process. She makes decisions about every aspect of her situation—about herself as a leader, about her group, and about the goals the group wants to achieve. The ability to make good decisions is an extremely important part of leadership in nursing.

Sound decision making is a basic part of organizing, teaching, changing, managing conflict, and evaluating. The nurse-leader who utilizes the decision-making process effectively will be able to engage in these other processes with greater ease.

The decision-making process may be viewed simply as making a choice, or—more comprehensively—as a systematic process that begins with a need or problem, and ends when an evaluation of the choice is completed. Viewed comprehensively, the decision-making process also involves making a choice, but only as part of a more extensive process.

There is a difference between problem solving and decision making. Problem solving is a less complex process, which is directed toward the solution of an immediate problem and often involves the trial and error approach. Decision making always involves evaluating several possible solutions and making a choice among them. Specific criteria are used to help the nurse-leader to differentiate among the solutions and select the one that is most appropriate.

TYPES OF DECISIONS

Decisions can be classified into two types—satisficing and optimizing. A *satisficing decision* involves choosing any solution that will minimally meet the desired objectives. An *optimizing decision* involves comparing all possible solutions against the objectives and choosing the solution that best meets the objectives (March & Simon, 1958, p. 140). Because identifying all possible solutions is often a difficult if not impossible task, a second definition of an optimizing decision has evolved. According to this definition, an optimizing decision is one that is made by comparing all *available* solutions to the objectives and selecting the one that best meets the objectives (Easton, 1973, p. 73).

Satisficing decisions are easier to make than optimizing decisions because the decision maker chooses the first solution he or she identifies that will solve the problem. This may or may not be the best decision. For example, a nurse who is shopping for a uniform finds one she likes and buys it. She has made a satisficing decision. When, an hour later she finds a uniform that she likes better, in another store, she learns the risk of making a satisficing decision—she knows a better decision could have been made.

Occasionally satisficing decisions must be made, e.g., in an emergency situation a leader must use the first acceptable solution that will solve the problem. However, in most nursing situations the nurse-leader will want to find the best possible solution. An optimizing decision is more likely to yield that solution.

JUDGING THE EFFECTIVENESS OF A DECISION

Two major factors are relevant to the potential effectiveness of a decision. One is the objective quality of the decision and the other is the acceptability of the decision to the group who will be affected by it (Maier, 1963, p. 3). Although more emphasis is usually given to quality, both quality and acceptance must be present to reach the most effective decision.

Quality

To determine the quality of a decision, several factors must be considered. First, what kind of input led to the decision? A good decision cannot be made unless complete, factual, relevant, and objective data is available to the decision maker. The decision maker must gather and use all the available data.

The behavioral characteristics of the decision maker affect the way he or she will deal with the data and use the decision-making process. The decision maker's perception of the problem will determine what data is collected. His or her personal value system may color the way the problem is perceived. In addition, the decision maker's ability to process data will determine the manner in which he or she compiles the data to derive potential solutions (Marriner, 1977, p. 40).

Another way to gauge the quality of a decision is to ask: Is the decision defensible? "A defensible decision is one that can be explained and whose every step can be recalled if necessary" (Bailey & Claus, 1975, p. 12). The decision maker must be able to state how and why the decision was made. To do this, it is essential to have adequate documentation. A written report can provide valuable information, especially after time elapses and details are forgotten.[1]

There are additional advantages for the decision maker who documents the decision. Documentation teaches the decision maker to be thorough in the use of rational processes and provides self-assurance about the decision. Further, the group and peers will respect this thoroughness. Documentation also can serve as a concrete method for demonstrating the soundness of the decision to anyone who is interested (Easton, 1975, p. 35).

Finally, to determine the quality of a decision, the results of the decision must be assessed. The highest quality decision is one in which the benefits outweigh the costs. The results also refer to how well the decision met the need or solved the original problem.

Acceptability

An effective decision must be of high quality, but it must also be acceptable to the group which is affected by it. If the highest quality decision is not acceptable to the group, its effectiveness will be diminished. In such a case, it may be preferable to choose a more acceptable decision that is not of the highest quality. When acceptability is included as a criterion for making the decision, a more effective decision will be made.

DECISION-MAKING MODELS

In the next section of this chapter, five decision-making models will be presented, all of which have been used by nurse-leaders. Each model will be described, and an explanation of its usefulness in nursing will be given. A practical example will follow in each case to demonstrate how the model is used in nursing. Table 8-1 shows the models in relationship to each other.

Kepner and Tregoe Decision-Making Model

The Kepner and Tregoe (1965) model consists of seven steps in the decision-making process. These steps must be preceded by a thorough problem analysis. The correct diagnosis of the problem or deviation is essential to success of the solution. The problem may be defined as "the deviation between what should be happening and what is actually happening" (Kepner & Tregoe, 1965, p. 20). Once the problem is determined, the first step in the decision-making process is to establish objectives that will provide direction for the rest of the process.

The second step is to classify the objectives according to their importance. Some of the objectives are essential and must be met; these are called "musts." Others are

---

[1] A clear explanation about how to outline a decision report can be found in A. Easton. *Complex managerial decisions involving multiple objectives.* New York: Wiley, 1973, pp. 51–52.

Table 8-1 Comparison of Decision-Making Models

Kepner & Tregoe (1965)	Bower (1972, 1977)	Easton (1973)	Vroom & Yetton (1973)	Bailey & Claus (1975)
1 Establish objectives	1 Determine what blocks goal attainment	1 Recognize need for change	1 Consider problem attributes	1 Overall needs and goals
2 Classify objectives as to importance		2 Diagnose the problem	2 a Determine type of problem	2 Define problem
		3 Identify affected interest groups; define decision objectives; assign numerical weights to objectives		3 Constraints and capabilities
				4 Specify approach
				5 Establish objectives
3 Develop alternative actions	2 Generate possible solutions	4 Identify all feasible alternatives	b Determine feasible set of alternatives	6 List solutions
4 Evaluate alternatives against objectives	3 Determine consequences of each solution	5 Predict and evaluate outcomes for alternatives		7 Analyze options
	4 Estimate likelihood of consequences occurring			
	5 Determine desirability and risk of each consequence			
5 Tentative decision is alternative that best meets the objectives	6 Choose best solution	6 Select a rule for choosing	3 Apply decision rules	8 Choose; apply decision rules
		7 Compute and make choice	4 Choose best alternative	
6 Explore tentative decision for future possible adverse consequences		8 Implement	5 Implement decision	9 Control and implement decision
7 Take actions to prevent adverse consequences, and make sure decision is carried out				
				10 Evaluate effectiveness of action

not essential, but would be helpful in making the best decision; these are called "wants."

The must objectives are all of high priority. The wants should be ranked in order of priority by the decision maker so that the more important ones can be satisfied before the less important ones (Kepner & Tregoe, 1965, p. 48). To rank the want objectives, the decision maker places a numerical value on each, giving the highest number to the most important objective. A 1 to 10 scale may be used or, alternatively, a number scale equaling the number of objectives. For example, if there are six want objectives, the most important one would be given the number 6, the next most important the number 5, and so on.

The third step in this model is to identify alternative actions, and the decision maker will want to develop as many alternatives as possible. In the fourth step, each alternative is evaluated against the objectives. The decision maker first determines whether or not each alternative satisfies the must objectives. If it does not, it is eliminated at this point.

The alternatives that do meet the musts are then evaluated against the wants. All alternatives are also compared with each other to see how well they meet the objectives. The alternatives are then rank ordered in the same fashion as the objectives. The alternative that best meets the objectives is given the highest score, the next best alternative is given the second highest score, and so on.

The score of each alternative for each objective is multiplied by the weight of the objective. The scores achieved are then added to arrive at a total score for each alternative.

In step 5, the decision maker chooses the alternative that best meets the objective. The alternative that meets all the musts and has the highest total score for the wants is called the *tentative decision*. Sometimes the tentative decision may involve combining two or more of the developed alternatives.

In step 6, the possible adverse consequences of the tentative decision are considered. The decision maker must estimate what problems could occur as a result of the decision, and how likely it is that they will occur. If adverse consequences are viewed as a low probability, the decision is accepted; if the adverse consequences are seen as a high probability, another tentative decision may have to be made.

The final step in the Kepner and Tregoe model is to control the effects of the decision by taking specific actions to minimize or prevent possible adverse consequences and to see that the decision is carried out. The decision maker carefully plans and executes actions to promote the acceptance of the decision and to ensure that its effects will be positive.

Usefulness   This model is useful for making nursing decisions when the decision maker has plenty of time. It is fairly complex and requires a good deal of thought.

One problem of the model is that there must be a large number of objectives—especially want objectives—and the decision is based on the want objectives rather than on the must objectives. In nursing there are few want objectives. Most objectives are musts.

Further, the consequences are not considered until after a decision has been made. Because of this, a different decision may be needed by the end of the process, or it may be necessary to begin the entire process over again.

Example This situation occurs on a twenty-two-bed orthopedic unit at a large metropolitan hospital. It is Saturday and Anne, an RN, sees that only an LPN, a nursing assistant (NA), and she herself are scheduled to work the day shift. Anne must decide how to make the assignments.

Using the Kepner and Tregoe decision-making model, Anne first establishes objectives, and arrives at the six listed below. She then classifies the objectives, defining the first three as musts and the last three as wants. Anne weighs the three want objectives (numbers in italic), giving the highest number to the most important objective.

1 All patients will receive holistic care.
2 The three team members will work within their job descriptions.
3 No injuries will occur to patients.
4 Patients will be assigned to a team member who has cared for them before. *3*
5 Team members will be satisfied with their assignments. *2*
6 Each team member will perform a fair share of the work load. *1*

For the third step in the model, Anne identifies three possible alternatives to solve the problem:

A The RN will pass all medications. The LPN and NA will each give care to half of the patients, and the RN will assist the NA with treatments.
B The RN will care for eight patients; the LPN will care for seven patients, and the NA will care for seven patients. The RN will pass medication for the NA's patients and assist her with treatments.
C The RN and the LPN will each care for eleven patients. The NA will assist both.

Next, the alternatives must be evaluated against the objectives. First, Anne compares each of the three alternatives to the three must objectives and finds that all the alternatives satisfactorily meet the objectives. Then the three alternatives are evaluated against the three want objectives. For example, alternative C most closely meets objective 4 (patients will be cared for by a team member who has cared for them before) and receives the highest score. Alternative B is considered next best; alternative A is least likely to meet the objective, and therefore receives the lowest score.[2] To evaluate the alternatives, Anne finds it convenient to use a table (see Table 8-2).

Anne then proceeds to the mathematical computation. Each score is multiplied by the weight for the objective, and then the weighted scores are added, as shown in Table 8-3.

---

[2] In this and other examples in this chapter, no attempt has been made to explain the rationale for the weights or scores that objectives and alternatives have been given. Each nurse-leader will evaluate them differently, based on the group and situation.

Table 8-2   Comparison of Alternatives against Want Objectives

| | | Alternative A | | Alternative B | | Alternative C | |
| | | Score | Weight × score | Score | Weight × score | Score | Weight × score |
Want objectives	Weight	Score		Score		Score	
Patient cared for before	3	1		2		3	
Staff satisfaction	2	3		1		2	
Fair share of work	1	2		1		3	
Total							

Anne chooses alternative C as the tentative decision because it received the highest score. She then considers the possible adverse consequences. The most likely problem would be that the NA may be less than satisfied with the assignment, but because Anne has worked with the NA before, she believes there is a fairly low probability of the NA being upset.

Anne then moves to the final step in the process—planning ways to minimize any adverse consequences of her decision. She discusses the assignment with both the LPN and NA, and helps them see why it is the best decision. Anne finds out which patients the NA knows, and plans for the NA to assist her with those patients. She selects for the NA tasks that will be helpful to her, and also challenging for the NA.

Bower Decision-Making Model

Bower (1972, 1977) has identified a six-step decision-making process (see Table 8-1). The process begins when the leader determines the need for a decision by identifying a block to some goal.

The second step—generating possible solutions—is the most important step in this model. Both the type and number of solutions are important. Bower's conceptual

Table 8-3   Computation for Tentative Decision

| | | Alternative A | | Alternative B | | Alternative C | |
| | | Score | Weight × score | Score | Weight × score | Score | Weight × score |
Want objectives	Weight	Score		Score		Score	
Patient cared for before	3	1	3	2	6	3	9
Staff satisfaction	2	3	6	1	2	2	4
Fair share of work	1	2	2	1	1	3	3
Total			11		9		16

framework guides the decision maker in generating alternatives. Bower includes three interrelated components in the conceptual framework: (1) the context of the decision-making process, (2) the character of the decision maker, and (3) the characteristics of the decision (1977, p. 83).

The context refers to the environment in which the decision will occur. Attending to the environment will aid the decision maker in identifying solutions that are appropriate in that situation.

The decision maker must be aware of personal biases, attitudes, and values, as well as of favorite approaches to decision making, because these will affect the solutions he or she will identify. The decision maker must try to be as objective as possible.

The characteristics of the decision, such as purpose, complexity, and consequences, must be evaluated by the decision maker since these have distinct effects on the possible solutions. For example, a simple problem should not have a complex solution.

Three additional factors influence the number of solutions the decision maker will consider (1) the number of solutions he or she can manage without becoming confused; (2) the number of people who are participating in the decision, and their abilities; and (3) the amount of time available for decision making (Bower, 1972, p. 83). These three factors are also related, since the more solutions and the more people involved, the more complex the decision making will be and the more time it will take.

The third step in the Bower model involves predicting all consequences for each alternative. Obviously, the more skilled the decision maker, the easier the prediction will be.

In step 4, the decision maker must estimate the probability of each consequence occurring. The decision maker guesses how often in ten times a consequence will happen, and then records the estimate as a decimal, e.g., .9 indicates that a consequence has a high probability of occurring—it will occur nine out of ten times.

Determining the desirability and risk of each consequence is the fifth step. The desirability or value of a consequence is determined by the extent to which it will achieve the desired goal, its lack of harmful side effects, and its efficiency and appropriateness in meeting the desired goal (Bower, 1972, p. 88). Risk is generally related to harmful side effects. A plus or minus sign can be used to indicate value or lack of value, and risk can be designated as high, moderate, or low.

The sixth and final step is to choose the best solution. Three guidelines can be used in making the choice: (1) choose the solution that has the most desirable consequences; (2) choose the solution that best meets the goals, with the lowest risk; and (3) if some solutions entail risks for the client, the decision maker, or the organization, choose the solution that has the least risk for the client.

Usefulness   The strengths of this model lie in its conceptual framework and the factors that relate to the generation of alternatives. The decision maker who considers these factors will select better alternatives and have an easier time identifying them.

Another strength of this model is that probability is considered. In other decision models it is possible to choose an alternative which has a low probability of having positive effects. When this occurs the decision may have poor results. In the Bower model, a possible decision is sufficiently scrutinized so that the results can be accurately predicted before it is implemented.

The major weakness of the Bower model is that it seems incomplete. Two of the rules for choosing the best solution are that desirable consequences and low risk to the client should be the basis for judgment. The third rule indicates that goals should be met. However, since goals and objectives are not in writing, this rule cannot be put into practice. This factor may lead to a purely subjective selection in the final step of this decision-making model.

Example The nurses on a psychiatric unit in a general hospital have agreed to begin peer review. They have decided to have two peers evaluate each nurse once a year. The nurses' goal is to have an effective, functioning system of peer review. The decision-making process has begun because the nurses do not have a method for implementing peer review, and the lack of a method is blocking their goal.

A committee consisting of three of the nurses has been assigned to develop a method. Roxie is the chairperson of the committee. The committee is ready to begin generating alternatives. Those they decided to evaluate are listed below.

1 The nurse being evaluated will select both evaluators.
2 The nurse being evaluated will select one evaluator, and the head nurse (HN) will select the other.
3 The nurse will be evaluated by two peers whose names will be randomly drawn.
4 The nurse being evaluated will select one evaluator, and the name of the other evaluator will be randomly drawn.

Roxie and her committee next predict the consequences for each alternative.

Alternative 1
A The nurse will select persons who will evaluate her very positively.
B The nurse will select persons who will evaluate her fairly.
C The nurse will select persons who will evaluate her very negatively.

Alternative 2
A The nurse will select a person who will evaluate her very positively.
B The nurse will select a person who will evaluate her fairly.
C The HN will select a person who will evaluate the nurse fairly.
D The HN will select a person who will evaluate the nurse very negatively.

Alternative 3
A The evaluators will evaluate the nurse very positively.
B The evaluators will evaluate the nurse fairly.
C The evaluators will evaluate the nurse very negatively.

Alternative 4
A The nurse will select a person who will evaluate her very positively.

B The nurse will select a person who will evaluate her fairly.
C The evaluator will evaluate the nurse very positively.
D The evaluator will evaluate the nurse fairly.
E The evaluator will evaluate the nurse very negatively.

The fourth step is to estimate the probability of each consequence happening. The committee sets up a table as shown in Table 8-4. In the fifth step, Roxie and her group determine the value and risk of each consequence, and fill in this information on the table.

Finally, Roxie must choose the best alternative. Alternatives 2 and 4 appear to have equal value and risk. Since the probability of alternative 2 is greater than that of alternative 4, alternative 2 is chosen as the solution for implementation.

Easton Decision-Making Model

The Easton (1973) model for decision making is a mathematical model comprising eight steps (see Table 8-1). The first step is the recognition by some individual of a need for change. The decision situation is assumed to be a problem, the solution of which will result in a change from the way things are. The person who wants the change to occur must call it to the attention of someone in power.

The second step is the diagnosis of the type of problem—or making explicit what the problem is. According to this model, most problems may be classified as problems of malfunction or obsolescence. That is, the system needs a change either because it is not working properly or because it is out of date (Easton, 1973, p. 57).

The next step in the Easton model has three separate parts. The decision maker must (1) define objectives, (2) place numerical weights or priorities on the objectives, and (3) identify the claimant groups, that is, the persons affected directly or indirectly

Table 8–4 Estimation of Consequences of Alternatives

		Probability	Value	Risk
Alternative 1	A	.8	—	LO
	B	.7	+	MOD
	C	.1	—	HI
Alternative 2	A	.9	—	LO
	B	.7	+	MOD
	C	.8	+	MOD
	D	.3	—	HI
Alternative 3	A	.5	—	LO
	B	.8	+	MOD
	C	.2	—	HI
Alternative 4	A	.8	—	LO
	B	.7	+	MOD
	C	.5	—	LO
	D	.8	+	MOD
	E	.2	—	HI

by the decision. It is important to identify these groups because certain characteristics or expectations of the group may determine what decision can be made.

The objectives are specific (measurable) criteria that will guide the decision maker in implementing the decision. The objectives are weighted in terms of priority, so that more important criteria will be met first if all the criteria cannot be met. The decision maker gives each criterion a number between 0 and 100, with the most important criterion receiving the highest number.

In the fourth step, the decision maker identifies all alternatives that are possible solutions, because the best decision can be made only when the best alternative has been identified.

Next, the decision maker predicts the outcome of each alternative and evaluates it against the weighted criteria. The analysis is most easily and clearly done in a tabular or matrix form in which criteria are placed on one axis and alternatives on the other, as shown in Figure 8-1. The decision maker ranks each alternative (giving it a number between 0 and 100) in relation to each criterion.

The sixth step is for the decision maker to select one of Easton's six decision rules with which to work. These are listed below.

1 Establish a standard of acceptability for every decision criterion. Reject any alternative with scores that fail to meet or exceed standards.

2 Establish standards of acceptability for every criterion except the *one* judged most important. Reject every alternative with scores on the nonreserved criteria that fail to meet or exceed standards. For those alternatives not so rejected, select the one with the best score on the reserved criterion.

3 Multiply each cell entry in the valuation matrix by the corresponding weight and add the weighted cell entries for each alternative (cross the matrix row). The alternative with the largest score is the best, the next largest, second best, and so forth.

4 Compute the weighted product of the cell entries of the valuation matrix by the formula

$$P_i = \prod_{j=1}^{n} (u_{ij})^{w_j}$$

The alternative with the largest P_i is the best, the alternative with the next highest, next best, and so forth.

5 Establish a dummy alternative with the scores 0, 0, 0, 0, and so forth as the worst possible alternative (absolutely repulsive on all counts) in a 0 to 100 space. Compute the deviation of all real alternatives in the valuation matrix from the worst case. The alternative furthest from the worst is best; next furthest is next best, and so on.

6 Establish a dummy alternative that represents the perfect alternative (for example, 100, 100, . . . , 100, in a 0 to 100 space). Compute the deviation of each real alternative from this perfect case. Select the alternative that is closest to perfection as the best, next closest, second best, and so on.[3]

[3] A. Easton. *Complex managerial decisions involving multiple objectives.* New York: Wiley, 1973. Reprinted by permission.

The seventh step in the model involves the mathematical computation and selection of the best alternative, based on the decision rule chosen. Finally, the decision is implemented. The decision maker takes responsibility for seeing that the decision is carried out as planned.

Usefulness The Easton model is applicable in many nursing situations. The identification of claimant groups is one strength of the model. Another strength is the attempt at objectivity that a mathematical model affords. (The numerical estimates are subjective estimates; therefore, the model is not completely objective.)

Because the Easton model assumes that all decisions involve change, it cannot be used in some instances. In most cases, continuing with the present system is a possible alternative, but this alternative is not acceptable in the Easton model. Another potential drawback is that *all* the alternatives must be identified. This is a valuable procedure because it ensures that an optimizing decision will be reached, but it is not always a practical or possible one because of the time it takes to define all the alternatives. Finally, the mathematical nature of the model itself can be a limitation because of the time needed and the sophisticated methods that must be used.

Example The setting is a pediatrics unit in a large general hospital. The nursing staff has been using brand X disposable diapers for several years. These diapers are also used in the newborn nursery. There has been a fairly high staff turnover in recent months, and lately there have been more and more complaints about the diapers. Most nurses believe the incidence of diaper rash is too high, and that it is related to the diapers. Some nurses find the odor upsetting for themselves and visitors when diapers are sitting in waste baskets for several hours. Other nurses are concerned about the biodegradability of the diapers.

Easton's decision-making process begins when someone recognizes a need for change. When Sam, one of the nurses, becomes aware of the complaints, and indicates to the head nurse that a problem exists, the decision-making process has begun.

The second step is to diagnose the problem. Sam and the head nurse agree that the problem is dissatisfaction with the present diapers, and that a decision must be made. The nurse-leader, Sam, agrees to be in charge of the decision-making process.

Sam identifies the claimant groups as he begins the third step in the process. The children will be the group most directly affected. But Sam knows that all persons caring for the children, i.e., nurses, physicians, and family members will also be affected because they will have to use a different diaper. Their feelings will therefore have to be considered.

Other groups will be affected indirectly by the decision. The newborn nursery staff may be forced by the administration to use the same diaper that the pediatrics unit selects. The purchasing department will also be affected if they must order another product.

Sam next establishes objectives for the decision and places numerical weights, or priorities (numbers in italic), on them.

1 Diaper rash, attributable to the diaper, will not occur. *100*
2 Cost to the hospital will be low. *80*

Alternatives

	1	2	3	4
1	50	50	90	100
2	80	70	70	80
3	100	100	100	100
4	100	100	80	90
5	70	80	90	100
6	40	40	100	100

Criteria

Figure 8-1 Easton evaluation matrix.

3 The diaper will be ecologically safe. *70*
4 Use of the diaper will be mechanically safe for the child. *100*
5 The diaper will fit securely. *80*
6 Disposal of the diapers will be convenient and odor-free. *70*

Since Sam knows that he must identify all the feasible alternatives (step 4), he calls a staff meeting to assist him in this process. The alternatives identified are listed below.

1 Brand Y disposable diapers, which are similar to brand X, but are biodegradable
2 Brand Z disposable diapers with elastic legs
3 Cloth diapers with plastic pants
4 Cloth diapers with no plastic pants

To complete step 5, Sam then sets up a matrix to evaluate the alternatives against the criteria (see Figure 8-1). Sam next selects a rule for choosing (step 6). He selects rule 3 because he finds it the quickest and most convenient. The computations are shown in Figure 8-2.

Alternative 4 has the highest score, which indicates that it best meets the criteria. As a result, the decision Sam makes is to change to the use of cloth diapers without plastic pants.

The last step in the decision-making process is to implement the decision. Sam must now work with the head nurse and the hospital administration to order cloth diapers and begin using them. Sam will have to carefully explain the decision-making process he used and why he believes this decision is best.

Vroom and Yetton Decision-Making Model

The Vroom and Yetton (1973) model for decision making has an approach that differs from the other models. This model is designed for a leader who wishes to determine what leadership style to use when making a decision. Before beginning the decision-making process the leader recognizes that there are five possible approaches available

Alternatives

		1	2	3	4
1	100	5,000	5,000	9,000	10,000
2	80	6,400	5,600	5,600	6,400
3	70	7,000	7,000	7,000	7,000
4	100	10,000	10,000	8,000	9,000
5	80	5,600	6,400	7,200	8,000
6	70	2,800	2,800	7,000	7,000
Total		36,800	36,800	43,800	47,400

(left axis label: Criteria with Weights)

Figure 8-2 Rule 3 computation.

for use with a group and five additional approaches for use in individual decision making[4] (see Table 8-5). The leader must determine which of the approaches, or decision methods is best for the decision he must make.

To decide which of the decision methods to use, the decision maker begins the process. The first step is to consider the eight problem attributes (see Table 8-6). The first attribute is the importance of the quality of the decision. Quality refers to the effects, or outcome, of the decision in relation to the goals for the decision (Vroom & Yetton, 1973, p. 21). Solutions that will produce the same effects should be valued equally, and it should not matter how the solution is reached.

The next two attributes involve the extent to which both leader and group have the needed information to reach a high-quality decision, i.e., information about possible solutions and their quality. The leader may have a great deal of information and expertise, while the group does not, or vice versa.

The fourth attribute concerns the extent to which the problem is structured. A structured problem has known solutions, or else the methods for identifying and evaluating potential solutions are known (Vroom & Yetton, 1973, p. 25).

The fifth attribute concerns the degree to which acceptance of the decision by the group members is critical to the effective implementation of the decision. Usually, a decision must be accepted by the group members, or it will not be implemented.

The leader must also determine in advance whether an autocratic decision is likely to be accepted by the group. The leader must predict how the group would deal with a solution that the leader confronts them with. Generally, group acceptance is related to the solution rather than to the autocratic decision (Vroom & Yetton, 1973, p. 28); the leader must therefore assess the group well in order to predict their individual and collective responses.

The seventh attribute is the degree to which the group members are motivated to

[4] The model, however, deals exclusively with the group problem situation.

Table 8-5   Decision Methods for Group and Individual Problems

Group problems	Individual problems
A1 You solve the problem or make the decision yourself, using information available to you at the time.	**A1** You solve the problem or make the decision yourself, using information available to you at the time.
A11 You obtain the necessary information from your subordinates, then decide the solution to the problem yourself. You may or may not tell your subordinates what the problem is in getting the information from them. The role played by your subordinates in making the decision is clearly one of providing the necessary information to you, rather than generating or evaluating alternative solutions.	**A11** You obtain the necessary information from your subordinates, then decide on the solutions to the problem yourself. You may or may not tell the subordinate what the problem is in getting the information from him. His role in making the decision is clearly one of providing the necessary information to you, rather than generating or evaluating alternative solutions.
C1 You share the problem with the relevant subordinates individually, getting their ideas and suggestions without bringing them together as a group. Then you make the decision, which may or may not reflect your subordinates' influence.	**C1** You share the problem with your subordinate, getting his ideas and suggestions. Then you make a decision, which may or may not reflect his influence.
C11 You share the problem with your subordinates as a group, obtaining their collective ideas and suggestions. Then you make the decision, which may or may not reflect your subordinates' influence.	
	D1 You delegate the problem to your subordinate, providing him with any relevant information that you possess, but giving him responsibility for solving the problem by himself. You may or may not request him to tell you what solution he has reached.
	G1 You share the problem with your subordinate, and together you analyze the problem and arrive at a mutually agreeable solution.
G11 You share the problem with your subordinates as a group. Together you generate and evaluate alternatives and attempt to reach agreement (consensus) on a solution. Your role is much like that of chairman. You do not try to influence the group to adopt "your" solution, and you are willing to accept and implement any solution which has the support of the entire group.	

Source: Reprinted from *Leadership and decision-making* by V. H. Vroom and P. W. Yetton by permission of the University of Pittsburgh Press. © 1973 by the University of Pittsburgh Press.

Table 8–6   Problem Attributes

A If decision were accepted, would it make a difference which course of action were adopted?

B Do I have sufficient information to make a quality decision?

C Do subordinates have sufficient additional information to result in a high-quality decision?

D Do I know exactly what information is needed, who possesses it, and how to collect it?

E Is acceptance of decision by subordinates critical to effective implementation?

F If I were to make the decision myself, is it certain that it would be accepted by my subordinates?

G Can subordinates be trusted to base solutions on organizational considerations?

H Is conflict among subordinates likely in preferred solutions?

Source: Reprinted from *Leadership and decision-making* by V. H. Vroom and P. W. Yetton by permission of the University of Pittsburgh Press. © 1973 by the University of Pittsburgh Press.

attain the overall goals of the group through the specific objectives for this problem. Here again, the leader must have thoroughly assessed the group in order to estimate their loyalty to group goals.

The final attribute concerns the amount of disagreement that group members are likely to have concerning preferred solutions. The leader must know whether or not group members are likely to have conflicts about solutions.

The leader uses the questions shown in Table 8-6 to find a simple "yes" or "no" answer with regard to each of the attributes. Following the model shown in Figure 8-3, the leader then determines the problem type. This is the second step in the model. The problem type is the number found at the end of the sequence in Figure 8-3 when the problem attribute questions are answered. The leader must next refer to Table 8-7 to determine the set of possible decision methods.

The third step in the Vroom and Yetton model is to apply the seven decision rules. The first rule is the information rule, which eliminates A1 from the set if the quality of the decision is important and the leader has insufficient information or expertise to make the decision alone.

The trust rule eliminates G11 from the set when the quality is important and the group cannot be trusted to make their decision based on organizational goals. The unstructured problem rule eliminates A1, A11, and C1 because greater interaction will lead to a better solution with an unstructured problem. The acceptance rule eliminates A1 and A11 when acceptance by the group is critical to effective implementation.

The conflict rule eliminates A1, A11, and C1 because if a conflict is likely, the group members must be able to discuss the conflict openly. The fairness rule is required when the quality is unimportant, but acceptance is critical. A1, A11, C1, and C11 are eliminated because acceptance will be greatest when all members participate. The last rule, the acceptance priority rule, also eliminates all methods except G11 when acceptance is critical and the group can be trusted.

When the leader applies the rules, he or she can then choose the best alternative—the fourth step in the decision-making process. If more than one decision method remains in the set after the rules are applied, the method furthest to the left is chosen (see Table 8-7). It is believed that the lowest number of man-hours that can be used for decision making is best.

A   If decision were accepted, would it make a difference which course of action were adopted?
B   Do I have sufficient info to make a high quality decision?
C   Do subordinates have sufficient additional info to result in high quality decision?
D   Do I know exactly what info is needed, who possesses it, and how to collect it?
E   Is acceptance of decision by subordinates critical to effective implementation?
F   If I were to make the decision by myself, is it certain it would be accepted by my subordinates?
G   Can subordinates be trusted to base solutions on organizational considerations?
H   Is conflict among subordinates likely in preferred solutions?

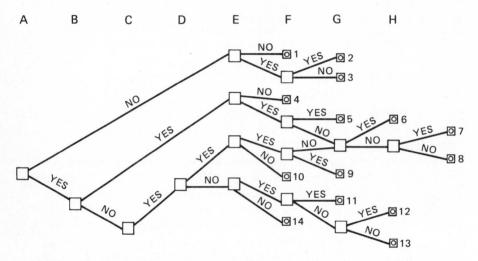

Figure 8-3 Vroom and Yetton's decision tree. The leader answers each question and follows the appropriate sequence. (*Reprinted from Leadership and decision-making by V. H. Vroom & P. W. Yetton by permission of the University of Pittsburgh Press. © 1973 by the University of Pittsburgh Press.*)

The final step in the Vroom and Yetton model is to implement the decision. The leader has chosen a decision-making method and leadership style that should result in success and must now carry it out, that is, use A1, A11, C1, C11, or G11 to make the decision.

Usefulness The Vroom and Yetton model is quick and effective for the purpose for which it was intended—selecting a leadership style to use when dealing with a group that has a problem. However, the nurse-leader who uses this model still needs to choose another model on which to base the decision that will answer the original need or problem.

A disadvantage is that the first step in the model requires subjective judgment; the decision maker has to estimate an answer to each question. Obviously, the better the leader knows the group, the more objective the answers can be.

Furthermore, the model is somewhat cumbersome because the nurse-leader using it must have the tables and rules with her whenever she wants to make a decision. Once the nurse-leader is familiar with the model, it is quick and easy to use.

Table 8-7 Problem Types and the Feasible Set of Decision Methods

Problem type	Acceptable methods
1	A1, A11, C1, C11, G11
2	A1, A11, C1, C11, G11
3	G11
4	A1, A11, C1, C11, G11*
5	A1, A11, C1, C11, G11*
6	G11
7	C11
8	C1, C11
9	A1, A11, C1, C11, G11*
10	A1, A11, C1, C11, G11*
11	C11, G11*
12	G11
13	C11
14	C11, G11*

*Within the feasible set only when the answer to question G is yes.

Source: Reprinted from Leadership and Decision-making by V. H. Vroom and P. W. Yetton by permission of the University of Pittsburgh Press. © 1973 by the University of Pittsburgh Press.

Example In a small, private nursing home, an 82-year-old woman has developed a deep decubitus ulcer on her coccyx. Nursing assistants have been giving most of her direct personal care. The nurse-leader, Jennifer, discovers that each nursing assistant is treating the ulcer in a different manner. Jennifer knows that a group problem exists and that a decision must be made.

Using the Vroom and Yetton model, Jennifer first considers the problem attributes. She answers the questions as follows: A, yes; B, yes; E, yes; F, no; and G, yes. From this analysis, Jennifer determines that she has a problem of type 6. When she refers to Table 8-7, she finds that the feasible set includes only G11. Consequently she can omit the third step in the model. Her best alternative is G11.

The final step in the model is to implement the decision. In this case, Jennifer would call a meeting of the entire staff during which they would discuss the problem of treating the decubitus. The group would then decide on a uniform method of treatment.

Claus-Bailey Model for Problem Solving

The Claus-Bailey model was designed as a systematic process for problem solving and decision making. There are ten steps in the model (see Figure 8-4), three of which are specifically related to decision making. These three—steps 6, 7, and 8—are called the *decision sequence*.

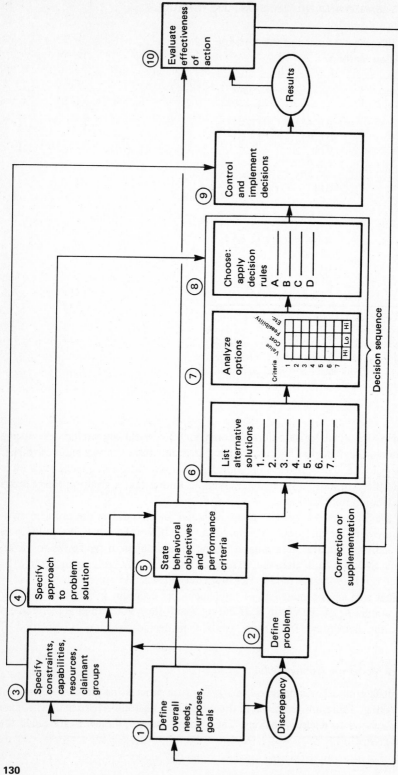

Figure 8–4 Claus-Bailey decision model. (*From J. T. Bailey & K. E. Claus. Decision making in nursing. ©1975 by Mosby. Used by permission of the publisher and authors.*)

The first step in the model is to identify the overall needs, purposes, and goals. These may have been identified before the problem or need for a decision arises, or they may be identified at the time the problem arises. The overall needs, purposes, and goals provide the framework in which the decision can occur.

The next step is to identify the problem—which in this model is called a discrepancy. A difference must exist between what some person wants and what exists, or between what is and what should be.

In the third step, the leader must compare the constraints and capabilities in the situation—the factors that will help in making the decision and those that will make it more difficult—so that the decision maker knows where to put the effort. In this step, the leader also identifies all the people, i.e., claimant groups, who will be affected by the decision in order to understand how they may view the decision.

In the fourth step, the leader must state the approach he or she will use. The approach refers to the assumptions the leader makes about decision making, and what factors will be treated as more or less important in the process.

Behavioral objectives for the decision are written during the next step. The objectives, which are specific expected outcomes for the decision, must also be divided into critical and noncritical objectives—those which *must* be satisfied, and those which are desirable but not essential.

The sixth step can be called the search step because it is at this time that solutions are prepared. The leader tries to find as many solutions as possible.

Analysis of the proposed solutions occurs next, as the leader compares each solution to the objectives and to other criteria that he or she may have identified, such as risk or cost.

In step 8, the leader chooses the best alternative on the basis of decision rules. These rules are directly related to the approach established in step 4.

The ninth step is to control and implement the decision. The leader will carry out the decision, being careful to do everything possible to promote its acceptance.

Finally, the leader must evaluate the effectiveness of the decision to determine whether it was successful, or whether it needs revision.

Usefulness The Claus-Bailey model is highly applicable to all nursing settings. Because the approach is systematic, the decision maker can easily go back and explain exactly how the decision was made. Moreover, the model has been designed so that the decision maker may choose to use the decision sequence (steps 6, 7, and 8) only, which makes it even more useful.

To complete the ten-step model is very time-consuming, and is therefore less likely to be used by staff nurses as part of their daily routine.

Example Sandra, a new nurse on a surgical unit in a large general hospital, has recognized a problem on the unit with patients who have had colostomies. She discusses her observation with the head nurse, who agrees to let Sandra make a decision. Sandra will use the Claus-Bailey model to guide her in her decision making.

Sandra knows that she must first define overall needs, purposes, and goals. She also knows that the hospital has a goal of providing comprehensive care for all persons. This implies that surgical patients need preoperative instruction because research has

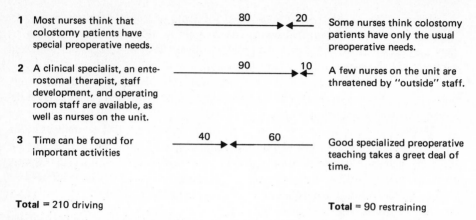

1 Most nurses think that colostomy patients have special preoperative needs.

80 → 20

Some nurses think colostomy patients have only the usual preoperative needs.

2 A clinical specialist, an enterostomal therapist, staff development, and operating room staff are available, as well as nurses on the unit.

90 → 10

A few nurses on the unit are threatened by "outside" staff.

3 Time can be found for important activities

40 → ← 60

Good specialized preoperative teaching takes a greet deal of time.

Total = 210 driving   **Total** = 90 restraining

Figure 8-5 Driving and restraining forces related to beginning a preoperative teaching program for patients having colostomies.

shown that such instruction aids in postoperative recovery. The goals Sandra defines for a preoperative teaching program are:

1 Provide the patient with information, so that he or she knows what to expect from surgery.
2 Assist the patient to have as speedy a recovery as possible.
3 Encourage each patient's participation in his or her own care.

The next step in the model is to define the problem. The discrepancy Sandra recognized is that patients who are about to have colostomy surgery are rarely given specific preoperative instruction about the surgery. She defines the problem as the lack of an organized, preoperative teaching plan for patients having colostomies.

Sandra next looks at the constraints and capabilities in the situation. She prepares a diagram as shown in Figure 8-5.

Since the sum of the capabilities is greater than the sum of the constraints, Sandra believes that the problem can be solved. Sandra also considers her head nurse and the clinical specialist helpful resources, and she consults with them frequently.

Claimant groups must also be identified. The patients and their families will be those most affected by a preoperative teaching program, and the effect on them is likely to be positive. Regardless of how the plan is established, the nurses on the unit will also be affected. Either they will carry out the program, or they will care for better prepared patients who will be more able to participate in their own care. Physicians and operating room personnel will also be affected because they, too, will have patients who will be more secure and knowledgeable about what is happening to them.

The fourth step is the approach. Sandra's approach includes the following assumptions: (1) patients should be actively involved in their care; (2) teaching is an important aspect of holistic nursing care; (3) preoperative teaching is most effective when there is a systematic plan for it; and (4) group teaching is as effective as individual teaching.

Sandra next prepares the specific objectives. Critical objectives are: (1) colostomy patients will be able to explain their surgery and know what will happen to them; (2) all colostomy patients will receive similar preoperative instruction; and (3) teaching will be individualized to each patient. Sandra added one noncritical objective: teaching will take 30 minutes or less.

The possible solutions that Sandra, in consultation with the head nurse and clinical specialist, identifies during the sixth step are:

1 Establish a videotape program of preoperative teaching for the colostomy patient that would be shown every evening at a certain time on the hospital closed-circuit television station.

2 Have the clinical specialist do all the preoperative teaching of colostomy patients in small groups.

3 Have an enterostomal therapist do individual preoperative teaching for all colostomy patients.

4 Develop a specific plan for preoperative teaching that would be attached to the chart of all colostomy patients and be completed by the nurse assigned to care for the patient.

5 Have nurses in the staff development department do all the preoperative teaching for colostomy patients.

In order to analyze the options (step 7), Sandra organized the data as shown in Figure 8-6, translating the objectives into performance criteria and adding a few other criteria that she felt were important.

Figure 8-6 Decision matrix related to the initiation of a preoperative teaching program for patients having colostomies.

	Benefit to patient	Consistency of teaching	Individualized to patients	Time	Quality of teaching	Availability	Cost	Score
1	(HI)	(HI)	LO	(LO)	MOD	MOD	MOD	3
2	(HI)	(HI)	(HI)	(LO)	(HI)	MOD	(LO)	6
3	(HI)	(HI)	(HI)	HI	(HI)	MOD	(LO)	5
4	(HI)	MOD	MOD	(LO)	MOD	(HI)	(LO)	4
5	(HI)	MOD	(HI)	(LO)	(HI)	MOD	(LO)	5
Ideal	HI	HI	HI	LO	HI	HI	LO	7

Sandra was able to choose alternative 2 as the best option because it had the highest score. Since no other alternative had the same score, Sandra did not need any special decision rules.

Sandra must now implement the decision. She will probably want to meet again with the clinical specialist to show her exactly how she arrived at the decision. She has consulted with the clinical specialist before, which will facilitate their working together on a plan for implementation. Because a new task is being added to the work load of the clinical specialist, other changes may have to be made.

After she has talked with the clinical specialist, Sandra will meet with the head nurse and the rest of the nursing staff to let them know what will be happening. Sandra must work carefully so that everyone will be satisfied.

Finally, Sandra will have to evaluate her decision. In 2 or 3 months Sandra should meet with the clinical specialist and the nursing staff to see how the solution is working. From her observations of the patients, Sandra will also evaluate whether they are better informed now than they were before the teaching program was initiated.

BERNHARD-WALSH DECISION-MAKING MODEL

After examining and evaluating the previous models for decision making, the authors decided that another model was needed—a quick and easy model that could be used anywhere. They therefore propose the Bernhard-Walsh model, which attempts to combine the strengths of the previous models while remaining simple to use. The model consists of the following six steps:

1 Identify the parameters of the decision situation.
2 Establish the characteristics of the ideal solution.
3 List possible solutions.
4 Choose the best solution.
5 Implement the decision.
6 Evaluate the results of the decision.

Step 1 The first step in the decision-making process is to identify the parameters of the situation. The parameters involve (1) the problem or need, (2) the people involved in the decision, and (3) the setting, or organization, in which the decision occurs.

The first parameter involves a clear identification of the problem or need. The decision maker must be careful to identify the real need, and not merely a symptom of a problem. A high anxiety level in a critical-care unit is not the problem, it is a symptom of some concrete problem, such as the deaths of several patients within a short time. Unless the problem or need is correctly identified, the decision that is made may not be the ideal one.

The second parameter is the people involved. This includes all those who are affected by the problem or need—whether they recognize it or not. Individuals may be directly affected, or their involvement may be indirect or peripheral.

As soon as the affected persons are identified, the decision maker should classify them according to their willingness to be involved in the decision-making process, and their ability to be involved in all steps of the process. Those who are willing and able should be involved throughout, while the opinions of those who are unwilling or unable should be considered, and they may be consulted during some steps of the process.

The third parameter, the setting or organization, must be considered by the decision maker because it will determine the type of decision that can be made. Organizations have a philosophy and policies which make certain types of care decisions possible and prohibit others.

For example, the philosophy of a mental health institution with a pain management center may state that patients need to be separated from their significant others for 2 to 3 weeks during behavior modification, and then follow up with teaching techniques for the significant others. In this instance, having open visiting hours would not be a feasible way in which to accomplish the desired behavior change. In contrast, a children's hospital philosophy may state that children should not be separated from the family; thus, rooming-in and open visiting hours would be mandatory.

Step 2 After the parameters have been determined, the decision maker should establish the characteristics of the ideal solution. The decision maker can accept input from the unwilling and unable group and take account of their feelings, values, and priorities. With the willing and able group, the entire group can suggest the characteristics of the ideal solution. The characteristics must be written as measurable objectives or criteria, since they will be used later to choose a solution closest to the ideal.

Several characteristics must always be considered. *Feasibility* is the first. A solution should be possible. If the solution cannot be carried out with the available resources, it is neither possible nor feasible.

The *value* of the solution should be considered, that is, the solution should have positive consequences. A related characteristic is *risk*. The ideal solution will not be dangerous to any of the persons affected, and will have minimal or no negative consequences.

The decision maker must also determine the *acceptability* of the solution. The persons affected must feel good about the solution, that is, they must like it and be able to call it their own.

Finally, the decision maker must also always consider *cost*—both immediate and long-term. Usually the best decision has a low-to-moderate monetary cost. The individuals and organization affected will almost always be happier with an inexpensive solution.

Step 3 Only after the characteristics of the ideal solution are established can possible solutions be listed. If this procedure is followed the decision maker is less likely to be influenced by his or her own "best solution" when establishing criteria.

Many factors affect the number and quality of solutions, including feasibility, time involved, and the skill and creativity of the decision maker and the group. Further, many approaches can be used for establishing solutions. All possible solutions can be listed, whether they were derived from brainstorming or on the basis of past experience.

Table 8-8 Table for Comparing Selected Solutions with the Ideal Solution

Characteristics of the ideal solution	Desired	Solution 1	Solution 2	Solution 3
Feasible	Yes			
Value	High			
Risk	Low			
Acceptable	Yes			
Cost	Low			
.				
.				
.				
Score				

Step 4 When the solutions have been determined, they must be compared to the characteristics of the ideal solution. This is most easily done in tabular fashion (see Table 8-8), especially if there are several possible solutions.

The decision maker first chooses an arbitrary scale, such as yes-no, high-moderate-low, or good-fair-poor, for each characteristic of the ideal solution and indicates the desired goal on the table. The decision maker then evaluates each solution against each characteristic and gives it a score on the scale. Each score on the table that coincides with the goal is circled, and a total score is recorded.

The decision maker is then in a position to choose the best solution. If one solution stands out as meeting the most goals, it is the obvious choice. If two or more solutions have the same total, the decision maker must make a choice between them. At least two methods may be used for making a choice.

One method is to reevaluate the total score for each solution by giving a half-point to any score that was midway, e.g., fair or moderate. If the total scores still do not discriminate a best solution, the decision maker might use a second method. This involves evaluating the scores of the solutions on the characteristic that he or she considers the most important. The solution with the best score on that characteristic would then be selected.

Step 5 The decision maker must then implement the decision, planning for all possible contingencies, so that the decision has the greatest likelihood of acceptance.

Step 6 Finally, the decision must be evaluated. The decision maker compares the results of the decision with the characteristics of the ideal solution to determine whether or not the decision is satisfactory. If the decision meets the characteristics, the decision maker continues with the chosen course of action. If it does not, the decision maker must begin the process again and find out where an incorrect or incomplete assumption was made. Once this is done, the process is continued, and the success of the decision is reevaluated.

Usefulness This model was designed to be used in many nursing situations. Each of the other decision-making models has its merit, and this model attempts to use the positive aspects from each, and remain simple. The model combines a consideration of the individuals involved with the usual steps in a decision-making process. Because of its simplicity, and the explicitness of the characteristics of an ideal solution, the model may be used by the nurse-leader in everyday decision making.

As with the other models, the element of subjectivity remains at the point at which solutions are weighed against the characteristics of the ideal solution.

Example Marilee, a primary nurse in a rehabilitation center, is caring for a primary patient, Clark, a 19-year-old paraplegic. Clark was injured in a car accident, in which he was the drunk driver. Marilee is an attractive, single, 22-year-old nurse. Since Clark came to the center he has been making sexual comments and exhibiting obvious sexual behaviors toward Marilee. This is the first time that Marilee has experienced such behavior, and she knows that she must make a decision about how to handle it.

If she were using the Bernhard-Walsh decision-making model, Marilee would already have begun the first step, because she has recognized that she has a problem in managing the care of a particular patient.

Marilee next considers the persons affected. She knows that Clark is primarily affected, and she decides that he is unwilling and unable to assist in the decision-making process. Several other health team members indicate that they are willing and able to help Marilee, so she consults with them during her decision-making process.

Marilee must also consider the setting. She knows that the rehabilitation center is greatly concerned about the sexual needs of patients, and that a variety of services and people are available to deal with these needs.

Consequently Marilee moves to the second step in the process and establishes her ideal solution. She first considers the required characteristics. The solution should be feasible as well as being helpful to Clark. It must have low risk to Clark, and also to her and the rest of the health team. The solution must be acceptable to all and of low cost.

In addition, Marilee establishes several other characteristics: (1) Clark's overt sexual behavior toward Marilee will stop; (2) Clark will openly discuss his sexual feelings and fears; and (3) the therapeutic nurse-patient relationship between Marilee and Clark will continue.

Marilee next lists possible solutions, after consulting with other nurses and interdisciplinary health team members, and getting ideas from some journal articles and books.

1 Marilee will discuss Clark's behavior openly with him and tell him that it is not necessary for him to try to impress her, that she likes him, and will give him good care.

2 Clark's psychiatrist will talk to him about sex and tell him what his sexual potential is.

3 Clark will be referred to a sex therapist for counseling.

4 Marilee will just ignore the behavior and avoid reinforcing it.

5 Marilee will encourage other young male paraplegics in the center to discuss sex with Clark.

Characteristics of the Ideal Solution	Desired	Solution 1	Solution 2	Solution 3	Solution 4	Solution 5
Feasible	yes	(yes)	(yes)	(yes)	(yes)	(yes)
Value	high	(high)	moderate	moderate	moderate	moderate
Risk	low	moderate	(low)	high	(low)	moderate
Acceptable	yes	(yes)	(yes)	(yes)	no	no
Cost	low	(low)	high	high	(low)	(low)
Stopping of overt sex behavior	yes	(yes)	no	no	(yes)	no
Discuss sexual feelings	yes	(yes)	(yes)	(yes)	no	(yes)
Nurse-patient relationship	good	(good)	fair	fair	poor	fair
SCORE	8	7	4	3	4	3

Figure 8-7 Decision table for the Bernhard-Walsh decision model, regarding a problem of behavior.

Next, Marilee prepares a table, so that she can weigh the solutions against the characteristics of her ideal solution (see Figure 8-7). Marilee chooses the first solution as the closest to the ideal solution because it gets the highest score.

Marilee must now implement her decision, so she arranges a time with Clark to discuss his sexual feelings and concerns. Marilee plans to be frank about her observations and share them with Clark. She also plans exactly how she will relate to him during their conversation.

Finally, Marilee will evaluate the results of her decision. She will compare what has happened to Clark's behavior, and to their relationship, with the ideal solution. If the results are positive, she will know that she has made a good decision. If the results do not agree with the ideal characteristics, she must begin the decision-making process again to determine what went wrong and to select a different decision.

REFERENCES

Bailey, J. T., & Claus, K. E. *Decision making in nursing.* St. Louis: Mosby, 1975.

Bower, F. L. *The process of planning nursing care.* St. Louis: Mosby, 1972.

Bower, F. L. *The process of planning nursing care.* St. Louis: Mosby, 1977.

Easton, A. *Complex managerial decisions involving multiple objectives.* New York: Wiley, 1973.

Easton, A. *Decision making—A short course for professionals.* New York: Wiley, 1975.

Kepner, C. H., & Tregoe, B. B. *The rational manager.* New York: McGraw-Hill, 1965.

Maier, N. R. F. *Problem-solving discussions and conferences: Leadership methods and skills.* New York: McGraw-Hill, 1963.

March, J. G., & Simon, H. A. *Organizations.* New York: Wiley, 1958.

Marriner, A. Behavioral aspects of decision making. *Supervisor Nurse,* 1977, *8*(3), 40–47.

Vroom, V. H., & Yetton, P. W. *Leadership and decision-making.* Pittsburgh: University of Pittsburgh Press, 1973.

ADDITIONAL READINGS

Archer, C. O., & Swearingen, D. Application of Benjamin Franklin's decision making model to the clinical setting. *Nursing Forum,* 1977, *16,* 319–328.

Aspinall, M. J. Use of a decision tree to improve accuracy of diagnosis. *Nursing Research,* 1979, *28,* 182–185.

Claus, K. E., & Bailey, J. T. Facilitating change: A problem-solving/decision-making tool. *Nursing Leadership,* 1979, *2*(2), 32–39.

Ford, J. G., Trygstad-Durland, L. N., & Nelms, B. C. *Applied decision making for nurses.* St. Louis: Mosby, 1979.

Grier, M. R. Decision making about patient care. *Nursing Research,* 1976, *25,* 105–110.

Janis, I. L., & Mann, L. *Decision making.* New York: Free Press, 1977.

LaMonica, E., & Finch, F. E. Managerial decision making. *Journal of Nursing Administration,* 1977, *7*(5), 20–28.

Marriner, A. The decision making process. *Supervisor Nurse,* 1977, *8*(2), 58–67.

Plachy, R. These are the elements of decision making. *Modern Hospital,* 1973, *120*(2), 97–100.

Taylor, A. G. Decision making in nursing: An analytical approach. *Journal of Nursing Administration,* 1978, *8*(11), 22–30.

Vanderwarker, R. D. The art of decision making. *Hospitals,* 1957, *31*(23), 36–38, 110.

Chapter 9

The Nurse-Leader
and the Change Process

Change is a phenomenon that occurs continuously in all living systems. Change is any alteration, regardless how slight or how major, or how large or small the object of the change.

Some changes are imperceptible while others are obvious. For example, changes occur imperceptibly in the human body as new cells replace older ones on the skin's surface; but in wound healing, the same process of cellular replacement becomes more obvious.

The nurse-leader must be knowledgeable about the phenomenon of change to function effectively. She is continually involved in the assessment and evaluation of her group and setting, and in the many factors that alter the way the group functions. Change is one of these factors.

Change may occur as a result of a well-defined plan based on an analysis of several options, or change may be made merely for its own sake. Change can be either planned or unplanned. Unplanned change is change that just "happens"—that depends on chance alone. In contrast, planned change is deliberate—a result of conscious decision making. Both planned and unplanned change affect group functioning and are therefore important to the nurse-leader.

The main focus of this chapter is planned change because this is the type of change the nurse-leader, acting as change agent, will be implementing. Suggestions for dealing with unplanned change will also be given.

PLANNED CHANGE

"Planned change is a conscious, deliberate and collaborative effort to improve operations of human systems . . . through the utilization of valid knowledge" (Bennis, Benne, Chin, & Corey, 1976, p. 4). Planned change is change with a purpose or goal, which is usually the improvement of a system through alteration. Planned change is also collaborative, that is, shared or participative decision making occurs. No one person plans the change; rather, all those who will be affected by the change are actively involved in planning it.

Target of Change

What is to be changed is often referred to as the *target of change*. Although many things can be changed, e.g., policies, procedures, and equipment, ultimately it is the person or persons affected—individuals or groups—who must change. The target, then, refers to the part of the person that must be changed.

There are three possible targets—the person's *knowledge*, the person's *attitude*, and the person's *behavior*. A change in knowledge is the result of successful learning, which can be accomplished through the teaching-learning process. A change in attitude may result from a change in knowledge when previous beliefs are found to be false or incomplete. A change in attitude may also result from a conscious effort to alter an attitude through value clarification or various types of therapy.

A change in attitude often follows a behavior change because the person's attitude and behavior must be consistent. When behavior change occurs before attitude change there is a resulting tension, which must be resolved. This tension is called *cognitive dissonance*, which means that a conflict exists between actions and beliefs. If the behavior causing dissonance is required or enforced, an attitude change must occur to lower the level of tension and allow the person to experience congruence between attitude and action.

A change in behavior may result from increased knowledge or from an improvement in skill acquired during the teaching-learning process. A change in behavior may follow a change in attitude or a change in expectations—whether self- or other-imposed—or may be the result of the normal growth and development process.

Hersey and Blanchard (1977) have conceptualized these three targets of change on four levels, emphasizing the degree of difficulty and the length of time required for change. This conceptualization shows how much more difficult it is to change an entire group's behavior than to change one individual's behavior. According to this model, a change in knowledge, whether in an individual or in a group, may occur with little difficulty and in a relatively short period of time, while a change in behavior will be more difficult and involve a longer time period (Hersey & Blanchard 1977, pp. 2-3). (See Figure 9-1.)

The Change Agent

The person responsible for changing the target system is called the change agent. Anyone can be a change agent. To be effective, a change agent must be familiar with the particular target system as well as the process of change. It is also helpful if the change

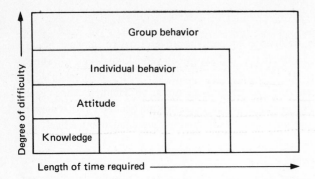

Figure 9-1 Four targets of change, indicating the increasing difficulty. (*From P. Hersey and K. H. Blanchard. Management of organizational behavior: Utilizing human resources, 3d ed.* © *1977. Adapted by permission of Prentice-Hall, Englewood Cliffs, N.J.*)

agent has support and acceptance from the person who has the greatest authority in the situation.

There are two types of change agents. The first is a person who is called in as a consultant to the group to assist them during the change process. Because this type of agent comes from outside the organization, he or she is called an *external change agent.*

The external change agent is usually a recognized expert about the topic of the proposed change or about the change process. The advantage in consulting an external change agent is that he or she can be completely objective about the situation, having nothing to gain or lose from the proposed change.

A drawback in using an external change agent is that it may take longer for change to occur, since the external change agent needs time to thoroughly assess the target. Further, the target group may realize that the external change agent will neither benefit from nor need to adjust to the change, so they may not offer their complete cooperation and trust.

The second type of change agent is one who comes from within the organization or group who will be affected by the change. This type is called an *internal change agent.* Such an agent has the advantage of being familiar with the policies, procedures, and politics of the organization. The internal change agent may also be familiar with the target group and may have already established a trusting relationship with them. The group is likely to view the internal change agent as one who will also have to adjust to the change, and they may therefore be more willing to support this individual than to support an external change agent.

An individual at any level of the organization can become a change agent. Although a high position in the organization usually guarantees power and recognition as an expert, it also means being removed from everyday detail. Workers at the bottom of the organization who will be affected by the change may view an internal change agent who comes from the top as an outsider and give such an individual less than their full cooperation.

An internal change agent who comes from a low-level position in the organization has the advantage of being thoroughly familiar with daily routines. An agent who is also a member of the target group may be in the best position to predict the effect of the change on that group.

Both types of change agents must develop a working relationship with the affected group. The basis of this relationship, as of any relationship, is trust. In many ways the change agent is a new member of the group, or a member with a new role; therefore, the group may need to proceed through the phases of group development.

It is important that expectations be clarified early in the relationship. What the change agent expects to do and what the group expects of the agent must be consistent. What the change agent expects the group to do and what the group expects to do also must be consistent. Mutually defining the expectations will minimize problems during the change process.

The Process of Change

Planned change occurs in a three-step process: unfreezing, moving, and refreezing (Lewin, 1951, p. 228). These three processes come from field theory, a method of analyzing causal relationships. Change, in field theory, is due to certain forces within the field.

Forces are directional entities that work in opposition to each other to maintain dynamic equilibrium. For every force there is an opposite force. Positive forces are called *driving forces;* they indicate the likelihood of moving a system toward a desired goal. Negative forces are called *restraining forces;* they indicate obstacles that decrease the likelihood of moving toward a desired goal.

Three possible situations result from an analysis of the forces within a field (see Figure 9-2). When the sum of the driving forces is equal to the sum of the restraining forces, a state of dynamic equilibrium exists. When the sum of the driving forces is greater than the sum of the restraining forces, change occurs in the desired direction. When the sum of the driving forces is less than the sum of the restraining forces, change occurs, but this change is further from the desired goal and represents a setback.

Whenever the forces in a given field are unequal, change occurs. The change may

Figure 9-2 Three possible situations that can occur with driving and restraining forces.

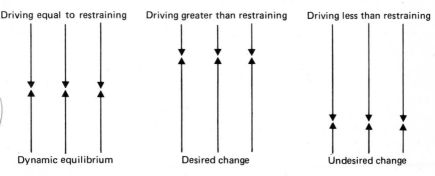

Driving equal to restraining   Driving greater than restraining   Driving less than restraining

Dynamic equilibrium   Desired change   Undesired change

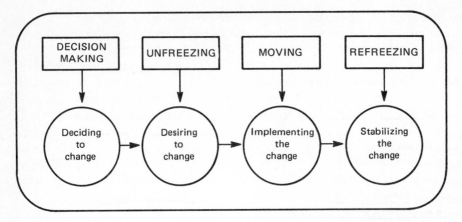

Figure 9-3 Relationship between the decision-making process and the change process.

be planned or unplanned. It is planned if forces are consciously and deliberately altered to move a system closer to a desired goal. It is unplanned when forces are altered by chance.

According to field theory, change involves three processes: unfreezing the present level of equilibrium, moving to a new level of equilibrium, and refreezing the new level so that it is relatively permanent (Lewin, 1951, p. 228). These three processes occur sequentially, with the moving phase dependent on the outcome of the unfreezing phase, and the refreezing phase dependent on the outcome of the moving phase.

The change process is closely related to the decision-making process. Decision making either precedes or occurs during the unfreezing phase. The decision-making process must have reached the point at which a specific option has been selected before the moving phase can begin. Once the change has been successfully implemented, the moving phase ends and refreezing occurs. Figure 9-3 shows these relationships.

Unfreezing Change begins with a *felt need*–a desired goal which has not been actualized. Any individual or group within an organization may experience a felt need. When an individual shares a felt need with another, unfreezing has begun. Either the person with the felt need or someone else may become the change agent.

During the unfreezing phase, present conditions are critically analyzed. It is assumed that conditions are stable, or "frozen." Once the present level of equilibrium is known, a plan to maximize driving forces and minimize restraining forces can be undertaken.

The goal of the unfreezing phase is to clarify what is and make the group aware of the need for change. Unfreezing attempts to bring about readiness for change by creating dissatisfaction with what is. The nurse-leader helps the group raise questions and explore feelings and attitudes about present conditions. When the group members acknowledge dissatisfaction with present conditions, they have begun to commit themselves to the change process.

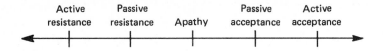

Figure 9-4 Resistance-acceptance continuum.

Resistance Resistance to change, though not inevitable, often emerges during the unfreezing phase. Resistance is any force which interferes with the change process (Lippitt, Watson, & Westley, 1958, p. 86). In a sense it is an additional restraining force. Resistance often occurs early in the change process because the present is known and secure, and any change will require time and energy. Even if the present situation is less than satisfactory, it is safe. Change, on the other hand, represents the possibility of failure and is therefore threatening.

Resistance can be conceptualized on a continuum with acceptance as an opposite (see Figure 9-4). Resistance may be either active or passive. Active resistance is overt and usually takes the form of outspoken opposition to change. Passive resistance is covert, yet it slows down implementation of change. Those using passive resistance hide their opposition from the change agent while attempting to sway others to their point of view. This type of resistance is more difficult to counter because the passive resistors may appear to go along with the proposed change while attempting to undermine it at every opportunity.

Some persons neither accept nor resist change. These persons generally appear uninvolved or apathetic. They do not pass judgment; rather they watch and wait to see what the change will offer when and if it is implemented.

Acceptance may also be active or passive. Passive acceptors comply with the change, but do nothing to influence others. They keep to themselves and do what is asked of them. Active acceptors enthusiastically support the change and attempt, through conversation and action, to convince others to support it. Persons who exhibit active acceptance frequently encourage and support the change agent throughout the change process.

The nurse-leader change agent must be careful to assess resistance as it occurs. Sometimes the way the change is presented rather than the change itself precipitates resistance. Vagueness about the proposed change may cause unrest in the group who will be affected. Therefore the nurse-leader change agent should be clear about what the proposed change does and does not involve. It is also important to show the group why the change is necessary and what benefits are expected from it.

The way the nurse-leader change agent uses time can influence the degree of resistance. If the announcement of the change can be made well in advance of the implementation, the group will have time to adjust to the idea of change, i.e., to become ready or "unfreeze," and resistance will be minimal. However, the time between the initiation and the realization or completion of change must be kept as short as possible, because the longer this time period the greater the resistance (Asprec, 1975, p. 22).

Resistance to the proposed change may actually aid the unfreezing phase as questions about the proposed change are raised. A clarification of what is, and what is planned, usually results from well-managed resistance.

The nurse-leader change agent who attempts to manage resistance must do two things: (1) allow the group to feel the need for change before proposing any options and (2) help the group explore options slowly (Lippitt et al., 1958, p. 75). Moving too rapidly to adopt a solution may mean losing the motivation for change, and settling too quickly on a proposal that does not meet the overall needs. The group must be helped to tolerate a period of uncertainty while options are adequately explored. If she allows the group to participate in the analysis of alternatives, the nurse-leader change agent will increase the group's commitment to change and decrease resistance.

Moving The moving phase is also known as the changing phase because it is during this phase that the change is implemented. The moving phase depends on the outcome of the unfreezing phase. If the equilibrium has been upset in a favorable fashion, i.e., driving forces exceed restraining forces, then change can occur.

Strategies for Changing The goal of the moving phase is to enact the desired change. For this to occur, the nurse-leader change agent must consider which strategy will best enable the group to successfully complete the change. Strategies are approaches used to influence a group to adopt the proposed change.

A variety of strategies may be employed during the change process. Three well-known strategies are the empirical-rational, the normative-reeducative, and the power-coercive. It is possible to use these strategies singly or in combination.

The *empirical-rational strategy* is based on two closely related assumptions: (1) human beings are rational; and (2) human beings follow a pattern of self-interest. From these basic assumptions it follows that people will change when they are shown that they will benefit from the change (Chin & Benne, 1976, p. 23).

The empirical-rational strategy is the oldest and most frequently used strategy. Its basis is in reason and intelligence. This strategy has frequently been used to secure funding for education and research that promise to improve the human condition. For example, human beings wish for health and a pain-free existence. Because they seek health, they are easily convinced to fund research projects that attempt to alleviate diseases. They also seek education in the form of explanations about the causes of disease and about measures to prevent disease. When they are shown that a program of immunization decreases the risk of contracting a communicable disease, people usually seek this intervention because they view it as reasonable.

The *normative-reeducative strategy* is also related to learning but is a more active strategy. What people do is determined by the norms to which they subscribe and the degree of commitment they have to these norms. Norms come from one's society, culture, religion, or family, or from other sources. Change occurs when commitment to some present norms decreases to a point where new norms can be adopted. Therefore, change resulting from the normative-reeducative strategy is more than increased knowledge, it is a modification of values and attitudes, as well as of behavior (Chin & Benne, 1976, p. 23).

The normative-reeducative strategy requires direct intervention by a change agent to aid in the unlearning and relearning process. The person who is to be changed must participate actively throughout this process.

To begin the process, the individual must be assisted by the change agent to view the needed change in the same way that the change agent views it. However, the needed change is *not* assumed to be merely a change in behavior; it is also a change in attitudes, values, and/or norms.

The individual and the change agent work actively together to produce the change. Behavioral science techniques are frequently used to help clients become aware of their unconscious values and norms, so that they may change completely to the new ones (Chin & Benne, 1976, pp. 32–33). During the process it is beneficial for the change agent to take the individual or group away from the location where the activity involved in the change usually takes place.

For example, when a visiting nurse association decides to change to a problem-oriented charting (POC) system, a change agent must be selected to assist the nurses to change their values and norms about the present charting system, so that they can accept the new system. The nurse-leader change agent may establish a series of classes about POC for the visiting nurses to aid them in unlearning and relearning. She will probably find a neutral location for the classes, or at least not the place where the nurses usually chart.

The beginning class or classes will focus on the nurses' present values and norms concerning charting. The nurse-leader change agent may use a values clarification or group therapy technique to help the nurses recognize their hidden attitudes about charting in general and about the particular charting approach they currently use.

Once they have defined their present attitudes toward charting, the nurses can devote the remainder of the classes to working with the nurse-leader change agent to educate themselves about POC, and to accept POC into their norms and behavior. The collaborative relationship between the nurse-leader and the nurses gives needed support during the uncomfortable process of unlearning, and provides positive reinforcement during relearning.

The *power-coercive* strategy employs the use of some type of legitimate power to force compliance with change. Very simply, those with greater power influence and control those with lesser power (Chin & Benne, 1976, p. 23).

The power-coercive strategy may be used by a person who is in a high hierarchical position within an organization to effect change that he or she, personally, feels is desirable or necessary. The group affected by the change is forced to comply, without having any input. They may simply accept the change, because they believe that is the way things are (Chin & Benne, 1976, p. 40), or they may put up strong resistance.

For example, if the census in a hospital is low, the administrator may decide to close a particular nursing unit. The staff on that unit are told that they will have to float throughout the entire hospital while their unit is closed. Some of the staff will comply without questioning, while others may be very upset and angry.

A change agent who uses the power-coercive strategy merely tells the group that they must carry out whatever change has been decided on. No input is allowed from the group. For example, the group may be told: "From now on, all diabetic patients in the hospital will be taught to use Ketodiastix. No other diabetic urine testing equipment will be used in the hospital."

Obviously there are many disadvantages to the power-coercive strategy; however, it may be combined with one of the other strategies to promote acceptance by the group.

In the example just given, the nurse-leader appointed as change agent could make the change less distressing for the group by using a combination of strategies. To do so, she should first approach the group to unfreeze them about the use of urine testing equipment. Next, she must tell them that the decision has been made to change to Ketodiastix—a power-coercive strategy that cannot be omitted. Then she can use either the empirical-rational strategy to get the group to see why the change is beneficial, or the normative-reeducative strategy to help them change their attitudes as well as their behavior. This combination of strategies is likely to facilitate the change.

Another power-coercive strategy is one that comes from legislation. When a law that affects health care is passed by a city, or state, or by the federal government, the nurse-leader will become involved, since constituents must obey the law.

If, for example, a state legislature passed a law stating that all public places must have clearly marked smoking and no-smoking sections, the nurse-leader change agent in a hospital would have to carry out the change. Since the group affected is so large (it includes all employees, patients, and visitors in the hospital), it would be impossible to have the entire group assist the change agent to carry out the change. The agent will be more successful, however, if she consults representatives from the groups affected, and uses either the empirical-rational or the normative-reeducative strategy, rather than just the power-coercive strategy, to facilitate the change.

Choosing a Strategy   In the course of the change process a relationship develops between the change agent and the group, which may determine which strategy is most appropriate. Who the change agent is in relation to the group also influences the strategy selected.

If a group views the change agent as an expert who has come to solve all their problems, it may initially seek a great deal of direction from the agent. However, as the group becomes more involved in the change process, the change agent may give the group less direction and encourage them instead to take on a more active and collaborative role. The change agent would then act to coordinate the group's activity to bring about the change.

It can be seen that, in the beginning, the change agent uses the power-coercive strategy, which is acceptable to the group at that time. Once the group is ready to collaborate, the change agent uses the normative-reeducative strategy, giving the group responsibility for the change and continuing to support them through the process.

If the change agent holds a higher position in the organization than the group affected, the change agent will have the power to use the power-coercive strategy. This is because the agent can control the rewards given to the group, e.g., job security, salary, and status.

If the change agent and the group are on the same level, the change agent has power only if it is conferred by the group. The group may allow the change agent to use power, but remains free either to comply with the change agent's directions or to remove the power from the change agent as it sees fit. Therefore, the change agent may have greater success in this situation by using either the empirical-rational or the normative-reeducative strategy.

Any change agent who wishes to maintain a productive working relationship with a group will need to use more than the power-coercive strategy, because a group that is told to do something is more likely to resist than a group that is involved in making a change. In fact, some group members will be angered by being told what to do by a change agent, and their relationship with the change agent will deteriorate. This will lengthen the time needed for moving. On the other hand, if group members are involved in the change process by a change agent who uses either the empirical-rational or the normative-reeducative strategy, they will be more satisfied with the change and will adapt to it faster.

The target of the change also influences strategy selection. The change agent whose target is knowledge can use the empirical-rational strategy. Those persons who see that an increase or change in knowledge is reasonable will engage in the project recommended by the change agent. The change agent may also need to use the normative-reeducative strategy, so that the group will value the new knowledge. The normative-reeducative strategy might also be used to create a readiness for learning.

When the target of change is attitude, the normative-reeducative strategy should be used, since it is specifically designed to deal with attitude changes. The empirical-rational and power-coercive strategies do not foster the development of insight, which is necessary for attitude change.

When the target of the change is behavior, any of the three strategies may be used because behavior is motivated by many factors, including knowledge, attitude, and adherence to authority. Some behavior change will occur following an increase in knowledge, which results from the empirical-rational strategy. Behavior change will also occur with commitment to new norms, which results from the normative-reeducative strategy. Finally, behavior change will occur when the power-coercive strategy is used and when noncompliance would involve great losses to the group affected by the change.

When selecting a strategy, the nurse-leader change agent must take into account both her relationship with the group and the target of change. She will be most effective when the strategy she uses is consistent with the overall goals of the planned change and does not jeopardize her relationship with the group.

With any strategy the change agent must allow time for the group to practice the change. Practice time serves as a trial period which allows the group to adjust to and experience the benefits of a new condition. The group can then evaluate their new knowledge, attitude, or behavior. When they see that their new knowledge, attitude, or behavior meets their desired goal, they will be reluctant to return to their former ways of thinking and acting.

Moving ends when the change has been fully implemented, that is, the desired change in knowledge, attitude, or behavior has occurred. When the target has been changed, refreezing can occur.

Refreezing The goal of the refreezing phase is to stabilize the change. The new knowledge, attitude, or behavior learned during the moving phase must continue to be practiced until it has become as familiar as the one that preceded it.

The nurse-leader change agent will know that refreezing has occurred when the group members consistently demonstrate the new attitude or behavior and verbalize about it positively, and when their actions and statements are congruent. Once it has been determined that refreezing has occurred, the group's performance should be evaluated periodically to confirm that the planned change is indeed refrozen.

The refreezing phase represents the end point in the process, indicating that the change has been fully accepted and internalized.

PLANNED CHANGE: AN EXAMPLE

A group of nurses on an oncology unit at a large hospital changed from team nursing to primary nursing 6 months ago. The change has been successful; it is refrozen, and the nurses are happy with their new roles.

However, the nurses are displeased with the change-of-shift report. They complain about the length of time the report takes, and about the type of information that is given.

Some nurses, in their frustration with report, have tried coming to work early so that they can read their patients' charts before report. That has not worked, however, because when they do so, they are enlisted to help the nurses on the previous shift complete their work.

Assessing the Present Situation

All nurses from both shifts go into the unit conference room for change-of-shift report, leaving only the nursing assistants on the unit with the patients. The nursing assistants pass fresh water to the patients while report is being given. The ward clerk and the nursing assistants can answer lights, but often patients wait a long time to have their needs met.

Report takes 30 to 45 minutes, and there is often a lot of social chitchat. No two people seem to give report in the same way, and the information is not presented in an organized manner. The Kardex is used, but not the charts or the physician's orders. Report about each patient is given to the entire group.

Unfreezing

This situation indicates that unfreezing has begun. A felt need is being expressed by most or all of the nurses for a change in their change-of-shift report. The *target* of the change is behavior, and the situation requires a *change agent.* Any one of several people could become the change agent: one of the nurses, the head nurse, a nurse from the staff development department, a consultant from another institution, or another individual.

In this instance, Cindy, a registered nurse on the unit, becomes the internal change agent. Cindy offers to get more information about different kinds of report, and the other nurses agree to work with her. The group has therefore given Cindy the power to be the change agent.

Driving and Restraining Forces   The first thing Cindy does is to analyze the driving and restraining forces. She finds that the nurses are indeed desirous of a change in the change-of-shift report, and she considers this a strong driving force. Another strong driving force is that the nurses have given her a leadership role in the change and that they all like her.

She finds two forces that are mixed, i.e., both driving and restraining: (1) some nurses want to socialize at the beginning and end of report, some want to socialize before, during, and after report, and some believe that socializing is only for after work; and (2) a few nurses believe they need to hear report on all the patients, not just on their primary patients, but most think it sufficient to hear report on their primary patients only.

The strongest restraining force is that not everyone on both shifts has the same patients. That is, a nurse on the evening shift may be assigned to a group of patients whose care is divided among different nurses on the day shift (see Table 9-1).

Table 9-1   Patient Care Assignments

	Day shift nurses		
	Sara	Jean	Cindy
Patients assigned	A	F	K
	B	G	L
	C	H	M
	D	I	N
	E	J	O

	Evening shift nurses		
	Tom	Laura	Carol
Patients assigned	A	B	E
	F	C	J
	G	D	M
	K	H	N
	L	I	O

Table 9-2 Analysis of Forces in a Situation Where a Change Is Desired for Nursing Report

	Force	Driving/restraining
1	Nurses want a change.	————————————▶
2	Nurses give leadership and power to Cindy.	————————————▶
3	Nurses want to socialize.	————▶◀————————
4	Nurses want to hear report.	———————————▶◀——
5	Nurses on different shifts have different patients.	◀————————————

Because of this, report could be confusing, and it could be possible to miss a report on a particular patient if all nurses were not paying close attention. Cindy decides that overall the driving forces exceed the restraining forces and therefore change can occur (see Table 9-2).

Cindy brings journal articles and other information about report to the unit, and she encourages others to consider possible ways of reporting. During unfreezing, Cindy and the group consider a number of options for report, and together they decide on the change: nurse-to-nurse report.

The Proposed Change   All the evening nurses will go into the conference room for report. The nurses from the day shift will then come into the conference room one at a time to give report on their patients directly to the nurse who will care for them on the evening shift. The report will be organized and given in the order of the information on the Kardex. The evening nurses may listen to the whole report or only to the report about their own patients.

When an evening nurse has received report on all her patients, she may leave the conference room. At least two nurses as well as the nursing assistants will always be on the unit to answer patient lights.

Resistance   Cindy met with some resistance from the nurses who wanted to socialize before, during, and after report because their social pattern was being altered. Cindy let them express their concerns and encouraged them to be involved in the choice of the new report method. She allowed plenty of time for them to become ready for the change.

One option that was considered was to have the nurses give report in the hall, but resistance occurred when several nurses thought that this procedure would be both confusing and complicated. Ultimately Cindy and the group agreed that it would be confusing. In this case, resistance resulted in the clarification of an option and ended positively.

Moving

To actualize the change, Cindy used the empirical-rational strategy. She met with all the nurses on each shift to explain the nurse-to-nurse report and exactly how to give it, and taught them what should be reported and how the material should be organized. She also discussed the mechanics of having two nurses on the unit while four were in report.

Cindy showed the group that the change would be helpful to them and to their patients for the following reasons: the nurse-to-nurse report is more personal; the day nurse will know who will take care of her patient during the evening, and the evening nurse can ask questions; and report will take less time because it is organized and because no socializing is allowed.

The group realized that the change was reasonable and, together with Cindy, they decided on a 3-month trial period for the new type of reporting. This would give them a chance to try out the new method and to be sure that they liked it.

Refreezing

During the trial period Cindy closely observed the nurse-to-nurse reporting, sitting in on each of the three daily reports several times. She answered questions, encouraged the nurses, and supported them in what they were doing.

At the end of the 3-month period, Cindy evaluated the results with the group at a full staff meeting. The results showed that everyone was enthusiastic about the new method. The reports were more complete and concise, there was less chitchat, and the nurses wanted to continue with this report method.

Cindy concluded that the change was successful and indeed refrozen. Furthermore, she was satisfied with her leadership role in the process—she had been challenged and had grown as a person because of the experience. She was willing and eager to be a change agent again.

HOW TO DEAL WITH UNPLANNED CHANGE

Unfortunately not all the changes that the nurse-leader encounters in her practice will be planned. What can the nurse-leader do to deal with unplanned change?

When a nurse-leader learns of an unplanned change, she must first recognize her own feelings and attitudes about the change, bringing them into the conscious realm where she can deal with them realistically. The nurse-leader should try to respond constructively rather than react defensively when confronted with unplanned change.

It will be helpful to all those affected if the nurse-leader can find out why the unplanned change is occurring. Often, when there is a good reason for change, the change is easier to accept. The reason for the change, as well as all its positive and negative aspects, should be analyzed. This procedure will lead to a more realistic estimate of the potential effects of an unplanned change. If the unplanned change appears to have more advantages than disadvantages, the nurse-leader should allow time for a trial period, and should also select a systematic method for evaluating the outcome of the change.

The nurse-leader must give support to those affected by the change. Any change causes an upset in the usual routine, but in the case of an unplanned change the group is likely to be more resistant and to have more difficulty adapting. The nurse-leader must do whatever she can to keep the group functioning effectively and to deal with the change.

REFERENCES

Asprec, E. S. The process of change. *Supervisor Nurse*, 1975, 6(10), 15–24.

Bennis, W. G., Benne, K. D., Chin, R., & Corey, K. E. (Eds.). *The planning of change*. New York: Holt, Rinehart, & Winston, 1976.

Chin, R., & Benne, K. D. General strategies for effecting changes in human systems. In W. G. Bennis, K. D. Benne, R. Chin, and K. E. Corey (Eds.), *The planning of change*. New York: Holt, Rinehart, & Winston, 1976.

Hersey, P., & Blanchard, K. H. *Management of organizational behavior utilizing human resources*. Englewood Cliffs, N.J.: Prentice-Hall, 1977.

Lewin, K. *Field theory in social science*. New York: Harper, 1951.

Lippitt, R., Watson, J., & Westley, B. *The dynamics of planned change*. Chicago: Harcourt, Brace, & World, 1958.

ADDITIONAL READINGS

Brooten, D. A., Hayman, L. L., & Naylor, M. D. *Leadership for change: A guide for the frustrated nurse*. Philadelphia: Lippincott, 1978.

Deal, J. The timing of change. *Supervisor Nurse*, 1977, 8(9), 73–79.

Grossman, L. *The change agent*. New York: AMACOM, 1974.

Levenstein, A. Effective change requires change agent. *Hospitals*, 1976, 50(24), 71–74.

McLemore, M. M., & Bevis, E. O. Planned change. In A. Marriner (Ed.), *Current perspectives in nursing management*. St. Louis: Mosby, 1979.

Mann, J. *Changing human behavior*. New York: Scribner, 1965.

Marriner, A. Planned change as a leadership strategy. *Nursing Leadership*, 1979, 2(2), 9–14.

Martin, W. R. *To cope with the current: Guidelines and activities for learning to deal with change*. Washington, D.C.: Association of Teacher Educators, 1974.

Olson, E. M. Strategies and techniques for the nurse change agent. *Nursing Clinics of North America*, 1979, 14, 323–336.

Rodgers, J. A. Theoretical considerations involved in the process of change. *Nursing Forum*, 1973, 12, 160–174.

Schwitzgebel, R. K., & Kolb, D. A. *Changing human behavior: Principles of planned intervention*. New York: McGraw-Hill, 1974.

Silver, C. The clinical specialist as a change agent. *Supervisor Nurse*, 1973, 4(9), 19–27.

Stevens, B. J. Effecting change. *Journal of Nursing Administration*, 1975, 5(2), 23–26.

Stevens, B. J. Management of continuity and change in nursing. *Journal of Nursing Administration*, 1977, 7(4), 26–31.

Tate, S. P. Automation of the health care system: Implications for nursing. *International Nursing Review*, 1975, *22*, 39–42.

Watzlawick, P., Weakland, J. H., & Fisch, R. *Change; Principles of problem formation and problem resolution.* New York: Norton, 1974.

Welch, L. B. Planned change in nursing: The theory. *Nursing Clinics of North America*, 1979, *14*, 307–321.

Zimmerman, B. M. Changes of the second order. *Nursing Outlook*, 1979, *27*, 199–201.

Chapter 10

The Nurse-Leader
and Conflict Management

Conflict is a part of everyday life. A conflict exists when two or more parties (individuals, groups, or organizations) differ with regard to facts, opinions, beliefs, feelings, drives, needs, goals, methods, values, and so on. *Anything* may be a source for conflict. Conflict produces a feeling of tension and people wish to do something to relieve the discomfort that results from tension.

Five characteristics of a conflict situation may be identified: (1) at least two parties are involved in some form of interaction; (2) difference in goals and/or values either exists or is perceived to exist by the parties involved; (3) the interaction involves behavior that will defeat, reduce, or suppress the opponent, or gain a victory; (4) the parties come together with opposing actions and counteractions; and (5) each party attempts to create an imbalance, or favored power position (Filley, 1975, p. 4).

Because of the discomfort that conflict produces, conflict has generally been viewed as a negative concept, and as a result many people try to avoid it. It is true that some conflicts, if allowed to continue, will lead to a deterioration in relationships, lowered self-esteem, and a decrease in production. However, conflict is a normal, unavoidable part of human relationships, and it can be a growth-producing process if persons learn how to manage it effectively. For example, conflict can promote change and innovation by challenging existing norms and practices; it can motivate people to reexamine themselves, their goals, and how they achieve their goals; and it can strengthen relationships. Without conflict, life would be dull and boring.

CONFLICT IN NURSING

Nursing has many potential sources of conflict, and nurse-leaders must manage conflicts each day. Conflict may arise between nurses, between nurses and other health team members, or between nurses and clients. Sources of conflict include patient care, health care issues, and schedules. The nurse-leader may experience conflict directly as an individual, or with her group. She will also experience conflict indirectly as an observer of conflict among members of her group.

Whenever the nurse-leader finds conflict, she must take it seriously and deal with it. She must be able to constructively and creatively manage the conflicts she is involved in so that she can set a good example for her group and for others. She must also be willing to assist others when they need help in conflict management.

The nurse-leader must be especially aware of conflicts among her own group members. Sometimes she will choose to let her group handle their conflicts by themselves; however, there are three instances in which she must intervene. If previously uninvolved people are being brought into a conflict, the nurse-leader must help them remain neutral if they wish. When a conflict disrupts the group functioning, the nurse-leader must assist with conflict management so that the group is not destroyed. Finally, if more time is being spent in the conflict than in the work of the group, the nurse-leader must aid the people involved to manage the conflict, so that quality patient care is not compromised (De Lodzia & Greenhalgh, 1973, p. 25).

RESOLUTION VERSUS MANAGEMENT

The literature on conflict discusses conflict resolution and conflict management, and a distinction must be made between the two. *Conflict resolution* implies a solution that completely satisfies all parties involved in the conflict. Rarely is it possible to satisfy all the needs of all parties because, to reach an agreement, some compromise will have to be made. It is therefore more appropriate to discuss *conflict management*, which implies a conscious effort to deal with the conflict and to control the problem. One does not guarantee to satisfy all involved, but attempts to meet as many needs as possible.

TYPES OF CONFLICT

Interpersonal Conflicts

Conflicts are of many types. Interpersonal conflicts are those which arise between two individuals, and these are undoubtedly the most frequent type, because people are constantly interacting, and therefore differing. Two staff nurses who disagree about the approach to use with a depressed patient are involved in a conflict, as are two children who want to play with the same toy.

Intergroup Conflicts

Intergroup conflicts can occur between two small groups, two large groups, or between a large group and a small group. A small group may be a family or a group of ten or fewer persons, or it may be a group that is small in relation to another group. For example, the staff on one nursing unit may include twenty or more persons, but it would be a small group in relation to all the other nursing units in a hospital. A large group usually refers to an organization or to an organized group of people that has many members.

Regardless of the size of the groups involved, intergroup conflicts have certain predictable consequences. Within each group, cohesiveness increases, but members become more task-oriented and less concerned with the needs of individual members. Group leadership tends to become more autocratic, but members nevertheless accept it. The groups become highly structured, so that a unified front will be presented to the opposition (Schein, 1970, p. 97).

In addition, each group begins to view the other group as an adversary, or opponent, rather than as a neutral force. Each group tends to recognize only its own positive aspects and only the negative aspects of the other group. Negative stereotypes begin to form and, as hostility increases and communication between groups decreases, it is easy to perpetuate the stereotypes. If the groups are required to meet, they will see and hear only those aspects of the other group that support their opinions (Schein, 1970, p. 97).

These consequences of conflict are both positive and negative. The increased cohesion and structure will probably increase production, but the stereotyping and hostile behaviors toward the other group are likely to be destructive to the persons involved. Conflict management strategies should therefore be used to ensure that the conflict will have a healthy outcome.

Personal-Group Conflicts

Conflicts between an individual and a small group or between an individual and a large group are called personal-group conflicts. In this type of conflict, an individual is at odds with a group. The nurse who does not finish giving her patients' baths before she goes to lunch will be in conflict with the rest of the staff if they believe that all baths should be completed by noon. This type of conflict is very difficult for the individual because he or she typically feels overwhelmed and powerless in the situation. The odds are all against the individual.

Intrapersonal Conflicts

Conflict may also be intrapersonal, i.e., within a person. The individual feels tension because of a disagreement within him- or herself. This conflict usually results from having to make a choice between two things of generally equal value, or from ambivalence about doing, or not doing, something. A nurse-leader who is offered a position in the pain management unit may experience intrapersonal conflict if she wants the new job, but also likes her present position on the psychiatric unit.

Intrapersonal conflicts may also result when a person is deprived of something he or she wants, but continues to strive for it. A woman who desperately wants to have a healthy baby, but who has had several spontaneous abortions and one stillborn child, may have a conflict about becoming pregnant again.

Management of intrapersonal conflict must come from the individual involved. Several options are available, but the individual must first decide what is most important, and then work to change the environment or his or her attitudes, or else use a systematic decision-making process to identify a solution. During the management process, the individual may also seek the assistance of others in focusing on the problem.

CONFLICT MANAGEMENT

Deutsch (1971) has suggested a number of variables that might be used to describe the course of a conflict. The *personal characteristics* of the parties involved—their values, goals, resources, beliefs, etc.—will affect the way they approach conflict. The *previous relationship* between the parties will also affect conflict management. Factors such as trust, respect, and degree of attachment will make them more or less committed to managing the conflict.

The *nature of the problem* that has created the conflict—its size, complexity, and significance—must also be considered. The *environment*, or setting, in which the conflict occurs can determine the type of interaction and conflict management that can occur. An interesting consideration is the *audience;* those who observe the conflict can aid or hinder its management.

The *strategies and tactics* that the parties use largely determine the outcome of a conflict. Finally, the *consequences* of the conflict for both the parties involved and the audience must be determined. Sometimes gains and losses may be more important than management (Deutsch, 1971, p. 37).

The variables discussed above are especially useful for a third person to use when evaluating a conflict or assisting other parties to do so. An assessment of these variables can help the third party by giving him or her insight into the situation. Presenting this data to the conflicting parties may also help them develop insight and come to an easier management agreement.

Approaches to Conflict

People use many different approaches to deal with conflict. The first is to *deny* the conflict. Denial may be conscious, but is more commonly unconscious. For example, the nurses on a unit may all be complaining about a particular nurse. However, when the head nurse asks that nurse what is wrong, and why she is not relating to the other nurses, she will say that nothing is wrong, or that she did not realize there was a problem.

Another approach is to *ignore* or *suppress* the conflict. The individual involved makes a conscious effort to forget about the conflict, saying, "If I don't acknowledge it, it will go away." This behavior may relieve the tension for a short time, but since the conflict still remains, the relief will be only temporary. The relationships involved will deteriorate, and the parties will continue to feel bad. This suppression of conflict, and its resultant problems, tends to make people think of conflict as negative and destructive.

A third approach to conflict management is the *win-lose approach*. A person faces a conflict by saying, "I'm going to win! I'll get him!" The intent is not only that he or she will win, but that the other person will lose.

It is risky to approach a conflict from this perspective, because one may lose as easily as win. There is no middle ground, and the opponent may be stronger and more aggressive. An interpersonal conflict involving a group that results in a vote is another example of a win-lose situation.

A win-lose approach often leads to a continuing feud or, in the case of nations—war. The loser is not likely to give up easily, and may keep coming back to attack. The loser will also be resentful and angry. The winner may feel guilty, but may not be able to renounce the winning position because of the effort it took to get there.

The opposite of the win-lose perspective is the *lose-win approach*. Persons who deal with conflict in this manner believe that they will always lose, and that their opponents will always come out ahead. They either deny that they have power, or give up the power they have. Such individuals either do not present their side of the conflict, or present it so ineffectually that no one listens. However, they always listen to what the opposition has to say.

The lose-win person may just be trying to please, or may think that the other party automatically knows best. Usually such a person has low self-esteem. Regardless of the reason for the behavior, the lose-win person will end up feeling hurt, used, and resentful, and the conflict will not have been managed.

Bargaining, or *compromise*, is another way to manage conflict. The parties involved agree to accept a solution somewhere between their two points of view. The bargaining approach is similar to the win-lose approach, because each party wants to lose, or give up, as little as possible. However, both know that they will not lose everything—as they might with a strict win-lose approach.

Bargaining is most likely to occur when one party has something the other wants. Most bargaining deals with money, as when an employee bargains with his or her employer for a higher salary. Bargaining may also involve other trade-offs; for example, a head nurse may tell a staff nurse who wants a day off that she can have it only if she will work on the weekend. The person who has what the other person wants obviously has the advantage.

When one approaches a bargaining situation, one must have an idea about the limits. A nurse bargaining for a salary must estimate how high she can go before the employer will refuse to hire her. Likewise, the employer who wants to hire the nurse must guess how low he or she can go before the nurse will decide not to take the position.

Mediation, or *arbitration*, involves the addition of a third, neutral party. A mediator is called in when other methods of conflict management have failed to provide an acceptable solution. When the mediator is selected, each party in the conflict presents his or her side of the conflict to the mediator. The mediator then makes a decision, or identifies a solution, that is fair to both parties.

Three conditions are necessary for mediation to work: (1) both parties must agree that some solution is better than continuing the conflict; (2) both parties must agree on the person selected as mediator; and (3) both parties must agree to obey the decision of the mediator (Hasling, 1975, p. 71). If the parties do not agree on these conditions, it is both costly and foolish for them to call in a third party.

The role of mediator is often uncomfortable, since the mediator often ends up being disliked by both parties. Nevertheless, if the conflict is managed, the mediation has been successful.

A nurse-leader may be selected as a mediator when members of her group are in conflict. Obviously, she must attempt to remain neutral and objective, and not become a party to the conflict as a result of the mediation.

Problem solving is a method of dealing with conflict in which both parties agree to work together for a solution. Problem solving is a creative, constructive approach to conflict management, but it is also a high-risk situation. Both parties must be open and honest in their communications, and trust the other party. All energy must be directed at the conflict or problem rather than at the other party. Because the parties work together, problem solving often produces the most successful outcome.

One final approach to conflict management must be considered—*withdrawal.* Withdrawal is not a generally accepted approach, but occasionally it may be the best one. Withdrawal is a costly decision for both the individual and the group, and for this reason, it should be a last resort only (Kielinen, 1978, p. 14). Only when differences cannot be managed in any other way should a person withdraw. If she makes the decision that withdrawal is her best solution, she can then go on with her life.

Bargaining and problem solving are the approaches most likely to produce a positive outcome. Thus, the nurse-leader will want to use them whenever possible.

Confrontation

When a nurse-leader, or any party who is involved in a conflict, is ready to deal with the conflict, he or she must inform the other party of this. This process is called confrontation.

Confrontation is a face-to-face, direct encounter with another person. It has been defined as an attempt to have the other person examine his or her behavior, in order to engage in more acceptable behavior (Johnson, 1972, p. 160). In interpersonal relationships, confrontation may be used *before* a conflict arises, to prevent a conflict from developing. However, when a conflict already exists, the confronter should also be willing to examine his own behavior, so that the conflict can be managed. The confronter does not want to put the other person on the defense, so he should be careful to let the other person know that he takes half the responsibility for the conflict.

When a person involved in a conflict confronts the other party, he is taking the risk of admitting that there is a conflict, and that he wants to do something about it. He believes that the reward of conflict management and a strengthened relationship is worth the risk.

The confronted party may respond in several ways. She could use any of the approaches described above, from denying that there is a conflict, to agreeing to problem solving.

Confrontation is an important part of conflict management, and as such, it must be engaged in carefully. The purpose of the confrontation is for both parties to recognize that there is a conflict and to agree to work on it. Consequently, the person who confronts the other party must select an appropriate time and place for the confrontation.

Ideally, the confrontation should occur in a private place where only the parties involved will be present, and at a time when they are relaxed and free from other concerns. Unfortunately, this is seldom possible in nursing; the nurse-leader must therefore choose a time and place as close to the ideal as possible. The nurse-leader should obviously not confront someone in the hall of the nursing unit, where patients, visitors, and other health team members will be present. Nor should she confront another person when that person is charting. Instead, she may confront at the end of a shift when she and the other person are the last ones in the conference room or locker room. Sometimes an appointment may have to be made. She could say, for example: "Could I talk alone with you for a few minutes sometime this afternoon, when we are both free?"

If the confronted party responds by denying that a conflict exists, the confronter may have to wait until a later time when the person is ready to deal with the conflict. If the confronted party responds by using a win-lose approach, the confronter must be careful not to respond defensively; he should instead indicate that he would like to discuss the matter further, but at another time.

When the party who has been confronted agrees that there is a conflict, and is willing to bargain or engage in problem solving, both parties can agree on a time and place for a meeting.

A mutually agreeable time should be selected, and the length of the meeting established in advance. If both parties know how long the meeting will be, they can plan their strategy within those limits, or else decide that more meetings will be necessary.

The location for the meeting is very important. The place selected should be a neutral area, i.e., away from the territory of either party. For example, the head nurse's office is not a suitable place for her to meet with a staff nurse with whom she has a conflict. A conference room on the unit or some other meeting room in the institution would be better.

Finally, at the time of the confrontation, the parties involved should agree on what resources will be accepted during the meeting. Resources include persons and material evidence or data. When a conflict exists about data, or interpretation of data, it is helpful for that data to be available at the meeting. If it is agreed that parties may have an advocate or ally present, the role of the advocate should be made very clear.

Strategies for Conflict Management

Balance of Power The first strategy that is of concern when managing conflict is to attain and/or maintain a balance of power between the conflicting parties. The purpose of power is to promote cooperation and collaboration in accomplishing a specific task (Claus & Bailey, 1977, p. 24), and if both parties do not have an equal power base, the situation can easily become win-lose.

Selecting a neutral meeting place is one of the first ways to promote a balance of power. Since one has more power in one's own territory than in another person's territory, the power is more equally divided when both parties go to a neutral location.

A nurse-leader who has conflict with a physician must use her personal power and resources to overcome the traditional physician dominance–nurse deference behavior pattern (Kalisch & Kalisch, 1977, p. 51). She may have to get past the physician-nurse conflict before she can deal with the specific conflict. Meeting outside the institution in which she and the physician work may help to equalize their power.

In a personal-group or intergroup conflict, power must also be balanced. One way of doing this is to have only one person represent each party at the meeting to manage conflict. Another way is to have a neutral third person present to observe. When an intergroup conflict involves two large groups, a small committee may represent each side. Obviously the group will want to select its most assertive and articulate members.

Communication Skills Persons involved in conflict management need good communication skills. Communication involves the sending and receiving of a message. Both parties must work to make their message as clear as possible, so that it will be received as it was intended to be received. Both parties must also listen actively, so that they will receive the correct message.

The communication should be an active, dynamic dialogue. Both parties should make concrete statements about their position and give concrete responses to the other party's point of view. When both parties make the effort to communicate clearly and effectively, they may find that the original conflict was generated by poor communication in the past.

Both parties must communicate assertively, that is, make their wants, needs, and feelings clear, while having regard for the wants, needs, and feelings of the other.

To use the language of transactional analysis (Harris, 1969), both parties should make adult statements, and behave as mature persons who listen to and respect one another. They are equals in the conflict—they have equal responsibility for causing it and should therefore share the responsibility of managing it.

Defining the Conflict Another important strategy is for each party to define the conflict or problem exactly as he views it. The two parties must then come to an agreement about what the real problem is. Until the parties agree on what the conflict is about, the issue will remain polarized, and nothing will be done to manage the conflict. For example, if one nurse-leader identifies a problem as "the nurses on this unit are lazy," and another nurse-leader defines it as "none of the nurses feel that they can work with you," a great deal of time may have to be spent defining the real problem.

Once the problem is identified, it must be stated specifically in order to make it manageable. "The nurses here are lazy" could not be dealt with very easily. The problem could be managed if it were stated as, "there is a lack of team spirit on our unit."

When agreement has been reached about what the conflict is, and it has been defined in manageable terms, all further discussion must center on that definition. Peripheral issues and past conflicts may not be brought into the discussion, since they will only distract the parties from managing the existing conflict and escalate emotions, thus hampering communication.[1]

---

[1] When the present conflict is managed, parties may mutually agree to deal with another issue.

Sometimes, especially with conflicts over values, persons cannot come to an agreement about the conflict. They may, however, "agree to disagree," that is, agree to allow the conflict to remain, but not to let it interfere with the rest of their relationship. Two nurses who have very different beliefs about euthanasia can still work together by accepting each other's viewpoint while making it clear that it is not their own.

Recognizing Human Needs Recognition of one's own human needs, and empathy for the other party's human needs, is another strategy. Each person knows how he prefers to be treated, and if he treats the other person in that way, more productive conflict management can occur.

Further, the specific needs of each party involved in the conflict must be considered when coming to an agreement or managing the conflict. For example, the nurses in a nursing home might have a conflict with the administrator about staffing. The nurses believe that staffing is insufficient, and the administrator thinks it is sufficient. Among their specific needs, these nurses might include time to complete their work and assistance in lifting, so that they will not be so physically exhausted and suffer from frequent backaches. The administrator's specific needs may relate to finances.

Rarely is it possible for all the needs of each party to be met. However, in conflict management, the goal is to meet as many of these needs as possible. If each party knows that the other party wants to meet the needs of both, more cooperative, constructive conflict management can take place. In the previous example, one possible solution that might meet specific needs of both parties would be to schedule the present staff differently.

CONCLUSION

Since conflict is an inevitable part of human existence, people must learn to manage it effectively. Various approaches to conflict management have been presented, and specific strategies for creative conflict management have been discussed that may be helpful to the nurse-leader. As more nurse-leaders—and other leaders—learn to use these strategies, conflict may come to be viewed less negatively. The following quotation speaks best:

> I was angry with my friend
> I told my wrath; my wrath did end.
> I was angry with my foe.
> I told it not, my wrath did grow.

> *Source unknown*

REFERENCES

Claus, K. E., & Bailey, J. T. *Power and influence in health care.* St. Louis: Mosby, 1977.

De Lodzia, G., & Greenhalgh, L. Recognizing change and conflict in a nursing environment. *Supervisor Nurse*, 1973, *4*(6), 14–25.

Deutsch, M. Conflict and its resolution. In C. G. Smith (Ed.), *Conflict resolution: Contributions of the behavioral sciences.* Notre Dame, Ind.: University of Notre Dame Press, 1971.

Filley, A. C. *Interpersonal conflict resolution.* Glenview, Ill.: Scott, Foresman, 1975.

Harris, T. A. *I'm O.K.–you're O.K.* New York: Harper & Row, 1969.

Hasling, J. *Group discussion and decision making.* New York: Crowell, 1975.

Johnson, D. W. *Reaching out.* Englewood Cliffs, N.J.: Prentice-Hall, 1972.

Kalisch, B. J., & Kalisch, P. A. An analysis of the sources of physician-nurse conflict. *Journal of Nursing Administration*, 1977, *7*(1), 51–57.

Kielinen, C. E. Conflict resolution: Communication–good; withdrawal–bad. *Journal of Nursing Education*, 1978, *17*(5), 12–15.

Schein, E. H. *Organizational psychology.* Englewood Cliffs, N.J.: Prentice-Hall, 1970.

ADDITIONAL READINGS

Gordon, T. *Leader effectiveness training.* New York: Wyden Books, 1977.

Hughes, E. Helping staff to manage conflict well. *Hospital Progress*, 1979, *60*(7), 68–71, 83.

Kramer, M., & Schmalenberg, C. E. Conflict: The cutting edge of growth. *Journal of Nursing Administration*, 1976, *6*(8), 19–25.

Leininger, M. M. Conflict and conflict resolution. *American Journal of Nursing*, 1975, *75*, 292–296.

Leininger, M. M. Conflict and conflict resolutions: Theories and processes relevant to the health professions. *The American Nurse*, 1974, *6*(12), 17–22.

Lewis, J. H. Conflict management. *Journal of Nursing Administration*, 1976, *6*(10), 18–22.

Mariano, C. The dynamics of conflict. *Journal of Nursing Education*, 1978, *17*(5), 7–11.

Marriner, A. Conflict theory. *Supervisor Nurse*, 1979, *10*(4), 12–16.

Smoyak, S. The confrontation process. *American Journal of Nursing*, 1974, *74*, 1632–1635.

Swingle, P. (Ed.). *The structure of conflict.* New York: Academic Press, 1970.

Tappen, R. M. Strategies for dealing with conflict: Using confrontation. *Journal of Nursing Education*, 1978, *17*(5), 47–52.

Thurkettle, M. A., & Jones, S. L. Conflict as a systems process: Theory and management. *Journal of Nursing Administration*, 1978, *8*(1), 39–43.

Veninga, R. The management of conflict. *Journal of Nursing Administration*, 1973, *3*(4), 12–16.

Watson, J. The quasi-rational element in conflict. *Nursing Research*, 1976, *25*, 19–23.

Chapter 11

The Nurse-Leader
and the Process
of Evaluation

Evaluation is a complex process used to arrive at a conclusion. The word evaluation, which contains within it the word "valu," involves determining value, that is, the merit or worth of something. Evaluation is a continuous process of deciding whether something is acceptable or unacceptable. The result is a value judgment. Each of us engages continually in evaluation, as we make judgments about our environment. When we complain that it is too cold, we are making a judgment. This may be an objective statement of fact—as, for example, when the numerical value on a thermometer indicates that it is below freezing—or it may be a purely subjective statement by a person who values warmth and notes its absence.

Evaluation is thought of as the final step in many processes. For example, the nursing process involves assessment, planning, implementation, and, finally, evaluation. Evaluation follows action; however, it also precedes, and in fact, directs the course of further action (see Figure 11-1). When the result of an evaluation is favorable or satisfactory, the behavior or action evaluated is usually continued. When the result is unfavorable or unsatisfactory, then the course or action is altered.

Evaluations may be done in many situations, but the purpose is always the same—to obtain feedback. Feedback may provide positive reinforcement when a system is functioning effectively or proceeding on a desired course of action. It may also help uncover problems or difficulties that need attention.

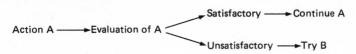

Figure 11-1 Evaluation follows and precedes action.

TYPES OF EVALUATIONS

Evaluations may be classified as formative or summative. *Formative evaluations* are process evaluations, that is, they occur during a process. The purpose of a formative evaluation is to determine which criteria are being met, and to pinpoint criteria that are not being met, so that energy can be directed toward unfinished areas (Bloom, Hastings, & Madaus, 1971, p. 61).

Since formative evaluations are conducted to determine what progress is being made toward reaching a desired goal, to be most useful, they should be scheduled at frequent intervals during the process. Nurse-leaders use formative evaluations during the teaching of clients to see what and how much each client has learned, and to help each one complete the learning process.

Summative evaluations occur at the completion of a process and are outcome evaluations. Their purpose is to determine which criteria have been met at the completion of a process. Summative evaluations tend to be more general than formative evaluations. This is because they evaluate the outcome, while formative evaluations seek out specific areas that need improvement. Discharge reports written by nurse-leaders to document the outcome of hospitalization by clients are examples of summative evaluations.

Evaluations may also be classified as normative-referenced or criterion-referenced. *Normative-referenced evaluations* identify the performance of an individual and compare it to that of an average, or normative, group. This type of evaluation may be used to determine the capabilities of a particular client in comparison to an average group. A standardized test is most often used. A nurse-leader working with children might use the Denver Developmental Screening Test as a normative evaluation tool.

Criterion-referenced evaluations identify the performance of an individual to determine if specific expected performances are exhibited. This type of evaluation requires a list of measurable criteria, a performer, and an observer. A criterion-referenced evaluation is used in the American Heart Association's (AHA) Basic Life Support Course. To successfully complete the course, one must demonstrate the specific behaviors or criteria required by the AHA.

Criterion-referenced evaluations are easier to use than normative-referenced evaluations because they depend only on the individual's ability to exhibit the desired behaviors. Normative-referenced evaluations depend on standardization, which is an involved and costly process. Without standardization, normative-referenced evaluations are purely subjective, and present difficulties for the evaluator, who must determine what "average" means.

Each type of evaluation has a variety of applications. The nurse-leader must be careful to select the type that is appropriate to the system or process she plans to evaluate.

THE EVALUATION PROCESS

To conduct an evaluation, the nurse-leader uses a three-step evaluation process. The first step in the process is *establishing criteria*. This is an essential step because the criteria are the foundation upon which a judgment can be made. The second step is *collecting data*, which provides the evidence to be used in the final step. The third and final step is *comparing the data* collected to the established criteria and *making a value judgment* about it. The accuracy of this value judgment depends on the appropriateness of the established criteria and the data collected, as well as on the objectivity of the evaluator. Each step in the evaluation process involves specific activities, which are further explained below.

Establishing Criteria

Criteria are statements of expected performance and must therefore relate to the thing or person evaluated. Three types of criteria are frequently used in nursing: outcome, process, and structure criteria.

Outcome criteria, also known as expected outcomes and discharge criteria, refer to the expected performances of patients or clients. Outcome criteria are written for specific clients in relation to specific conditions or problems. The outcome criterion states the expected performance in measurable terms, so that both the client and the other health team members can monitor the client's progress.

Process criteria refer to the expected performances of nurses and are written in terms of the nursing process. These criteria state the expected performances of the nurse in measurable terms. Process criteria provide a way to judge the care given to clients by nurses as a group. They may also be used to evaluate an individual nurse's performance.

Structure criteria refer to the expected performance of an organization. They include environmental factors, such as physical layout and safety features. Structure criteria may also be procedural, e.g., the standards used to evaluate the care provided by an institution or agency.

The American Nurses' Association has written and published standards for nursing practice that can be used as criteria to evaluate the practice of a single nurse or a group of nurses. The initial *Standards of Nursing Practice* (ANA, 1973a) are general standards that are applicable to all areas of nursing. The ANA has also drawn up standards for each of the major specialties in nursing, such as the *Standards of Psychiatric–Mental Health Nursing Practice* (ANA, 1973b), the *Standards of Gerontological Nursing Practice* (ANA, 1976), and the *Standards of Cardiovascular Nursing Practice* (ANA, 1975).

All the standards may be used in their original form to evaluate nursing practice or they may be refined or individualized to be used in a particular institution. For example, the standard, "Nursing actions provide for consumer participation in health promotion, maintenance, and restoration" (*Standards of Community Health Nursing Practice*, ANA, 1974, unpaged) could be used as is in any community health agency. Alternatively, in a particular community health agency, it could be spelled out as follows: "At the well-baby clinic, the public health nurse seeks input from parents regarding educational classes they desire."

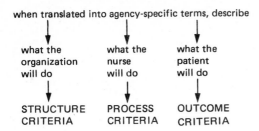

ANA Standards of Nursing Practice

when translated into agency-specific terms, describe

| what the organization will do | what the nurse will do | what the patient will do |

STRUCTURE CRITERIA | PROCESS CRITERIA | OUTCOME CRITERIA

Figure 11-2 How overall standards become specific criteria.

Well-written job descriptions provide an excellent source for criteria that can be used to evaluate nurses' performance. Job descriptions should list specific behaviors for which the jobholder is responsible, and the jobholder should be evaluated according to those behaviors. "Participates in planning, implementing, coordinating, and evaluating nursing care" is a statement that could be found in a job description, and that could serve as a criterion for evaluating a registered nurse.

Organizations such as the National League for Nursing (NLN) and the Joint Commission on the Accreditation of Hospitals (JCAH) that accredit nursing schools, home health agencies, and hospitals have written criteria for accreditation. These criteria may be modified for use by nurse-leaders in specific settings.

Any of these sources of criteria may be used by the nurse-leader to develop specific outcome, process, and structure criteria. By specifying the structure criteria, the nurse-leader is able to indicate what the organization will do to help the nurses to meet the process criteria. The process criteria indicate what the nurses will do to enable the clients to meet the outcome criteria. When using existing criteria, the nurse-leader must translate each criterion into agency-specific terminology and specify all three types of criteria (see Figure 11-2).

Whether the nurse-leader writes her own criteria or adapts existing criteria to her setting, she should keep in mind the characteristics of sound objectives. Well-developed criteria have the same characteristics as sound objectives: they are acceptable, attainable, simple, communicated, and motivational (Jucius, Deitzer, & Schlender, 1973, pp. 167-168).

An acceptable criterion is one which is a valid indicator of the expected performance. This means that the criterion is accurate, and measures what it is supposed to measure. For example, the apical pulse is a valid indicator of heart rate while arterial blood pressure or respiratory excursion are unacceptable criteria because they do not measure heart rate.

An attainable criterion is one which is realistic for the person who is expected to perform and for the situation in which the evaluation is conducted. This does not mean that every performer is able to meet the criterion every time but, rather, that it is at least theoretically possible for every performer to meet the criterion at some point in time. An attainable criterion for an adult undergoing abdominal surgery could be "ambulate without assistance." Not all clients in this situation will be able to ambulate immediately postoperatively, but they should certainly do so before discharge.

A simple criterion is one which is clearly and concisely written; it should not be vague or ambiguous. A simple criterion must also be specific. At first glance, a criterion stating that a "client will remain afebrile" may appear specific. But one individual may interpret afebrile as higher than 98.6°F, while another may interpret it as below 100°F or 101°F. Obviously "afebrile" is not a specific criterion and therefore not simple.

Criteria must also be communicated. Before any performance is evaluated, both the evaluator and the person expected to perform must be cognizant of the criteria and have the same understanding of the expected level of performance. The criteria must be communicated openly and clearly. If the evaluator and the performer perceive the criteria in a similar manner, the results of the evaluation are more likely to be acceptable to them. If, however, the performer has a different understanding of the criteria, or is unaware of the criteria, he or she is unlikely to accept the results of the evaluation.

Criteria must also be motivational, that is, indicate what is desired. A criterion should be stated as a positive, observable behavior or measurement rather than an absence of an undesirable behavior or measurement. It would be better to state the criterion, "soiled linen is placed in a hamper after use," than "there is no soiled linen on the floor." Both statements indicate the desired behavior, but the first is more positive and directive. Positive statements are more likely to motivate and guide behavior than negative ones.

Collecting Data

Once the criteria are established, the second step in the evaluation process—collecting data—may begin. The criteria indicate the type of data needed, the second step how the data will be collected.

Before deciding on a method of data collection, the nurse-leader needs to analyze her own feelings and attitudes about the person or system she plans to evaluate. Objectivity is necessary in utilizing any data-collecting instrument. The evaluator may perceive either what he or she wishes to see or what is actually present. An evalaution is only as objective as the evaluator who conducts it.

Methods of Data Collection A *checklist* is an instrument commonly used to collect data. It is easily constructed and simple to use. The checklist usually contains a list of the desired criteria, with spaces or boxes to indicate if each criterion is accomplished (see Figure 11-3).

Figure 11-3 Example of a checklist.

		YES	NO
1	Washes hands before gowning	☑	☐
2	Selects clean gown from cabinet	☑	☐
3	Closes door immediately after entering room	☐	☑

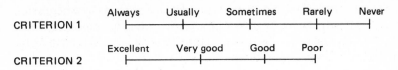

Figure 11-4 Examples of rating scales.

A disadvantage of this method is that it may be difficult to list each specific criterion in a complex process, or else the list may be too long. Also, a checklist usually represents a single performance, which may or may not be a typical performance of the person being evaluated.

A second type of data-collecting instrument is the *rating scale*. The rating scale is similar to the checklist in its simplicity and usability. It, too, is composed of a list of criteria and a section for recording if the criteria are met. The rating scale, however, calls for a judgment about how well, or how often, the criterion is met (see Figure 11-4).

Any number of words may be used on the scale. Some scales use numbers instead of words, while others use a combination of words and numbers.

The rating scale requires more interpretation by the evaluator than the checklist, and more than one observation of performance is generally needed. It is helpful to both the evaluator and the person evaluated if operational definitions are supplied for the words used on the scale. For example, "usually" might be defined as three out of four times, "sometimes" as two out of four times, and "rarely" as once in four times.

In order to maximize the usefulness of the rating scale, another way of constructing it has been suggested. Using this method, criteria are written for each level of performance (see Figure 11-5). By specifying each level of performance, the scale can be interpreted by every evaluator in a similar manner. The levels represented on the scale may also serve as a guide to the person evaluated because the scale indicates specifically the best behavior. For example, a desirable behavior which is expected of nurses is to involve the client and the client's significant others in the planning of care. A particular nurse might talk to her clients and show interest in them, and in their families and friends. Therefore, when this nurse is evaluated on the criterion stating that "the nurse involves the client and significant others in the planning of care," she may be surprised to find herself rated as "poor," or as "2" on a simple 0 to 5 scale. If, how-

Figure 11-5 Example of a performance rating scale.

CRITERION 1: Involves client and significant others in planning of care

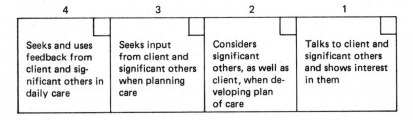

ever, she has access to the scale in Figure 11-5, she will be able to evaluate her performance realistically, and increase her awareness of what the criterion means.

A third type of data-collecting instrument is the *anecdotal note*. This method differs from the other methods in both form and use. The evaluator using this method records events as they occur, or as soon as possible afterward. A complete and objective description of an event is recorded in narrative form and the setting in which the event occurred is described in sufficient detail to give meaning to the event. The event chosen is either representative of typical behavior or is significant because it is markedly different from the person's usual behavior. A good anecdotal note would also include an interpretation by the evaluator, which is separated from the description of the event and labeled as an interpretation (Thorndike & Hagen, 1969, p. 486).

The following is an example of an anecdotal note:

Re:Sara Larson, graduate nurse   8–23–80

Sara was assigned to provide care for four patients today. One was Mrs. J. D., a 30-year-old woman who had major abdominal surgery yesterday. Sara gave Mrs. J. D. a basin of water, told her to bathe herself, and left the room. The patient did give herself a bath, but was quite exhausted afterwards.

Interpretation: It is unusual to have a patient, on the first postoperative day, completely do her own bath. Ordinarily, a nurse would provide assistance or at least stay with the patient. Sara was informed of this.

K. Cook, RN (Sig.)

Before a judgment can be made, several anecdotal notes must be compiled to determine a pattern of behavior. Anecdotal notes are useful to the nurse-leader who must evaluate group members. They can serve as an ongoing document of events considered important by the nurse-leader, and they are much more accurate than recall, which may take place days or months after the incident. It is best to write anecdotal notes on a regular basis, daily or weekly, and compile the information at a specified interval.

The *process recording* is another data collection tool. Process recordings include verbatim interactions, usually between client and nurse, and an interpretation of the interactions, or a rationale, provided by the recorder. Frequently, a third section is included, which provides theoretical or background material viewed as relevant (see Table 11-1).

The process recording is useful for analysis of communication. It is most often used when students or new graduates are learning to communicate with particular clients. It is also a helpful tool for self-evaluation. One problem with the process recording is that conversation must be recalled, and this is a difficult task.[1] It is possible to alter the meaning of statements by omission, whether intentional or unintentional. The process recording is used infrequently because of the subjectivity involved.

[1] A tape recorder can be used, but its presence may affect the communication between nurse and client. Permission from the client must also be obtained before recording a conversation.

Table 11-1   Example of a Process Recording

Interaction	Interpretation rationale	Theoretical base
Nurse: How are you feeling today?	Since the primary nurse had said that he seemed depressed, I wanted to find out from him.	Open-ended questions allow the patient to direct the conversation.
Patient: Rotten.	He looked tired and depressed.	
Nurse: Rotten?	I wanted him to explain what he meant.	Reflective technique helps the patient to elaborate on his feelings.
Patient: Yes. I didn't sleep a wink all night.	Now he sounded angry.	

Compare and Make a Judgment

Once the data has been gathered, it is compiled into some form. If a checklist or rating scale was used, a score is usually determined. If another method has been used, the data should be placed in chronological order, and note may be made regarding significant data. The number of positive, negative, and neutral incidents might also be noted. The purpose of compiling the data is to make it usable in the final step of the evaluation process.

After the data is collected and compiled in an organized, usable manner, the nurse-leader compares it with the established criteria. Judgment is used to determine if criteria are met, and the extent to which each criterion is met.

When comparing the data to the established criteria and making a judgment, it is important to consider the source of the data. Does the data come from a direct or an indirect source? Direct data is collected by observing the actual performance or event being evaluated. Indirect data is collected by assessing the product or outcome of the event, or from written records that document the event.

The accuracy of direct data depends on the perception and objectivity of the evaluator. Usually direct data is an accurate representation of what has occurred. The accuracy of indirect data is more questionable, since several variables may influence the product or outcome of a process.

For example, what is seen as the result of a particular action may, in fact, be the result of some other action or a consequence of chance. Furthermore, written records contain reports by persons whose credibility may be assumed but cannot be proven. Critical factors may be inadvertently omitted in a written record. From the legal standpoint, the following assumption is made: if it is not charted, it was not done (Bishop, 1975, p. 11).

A nurse-leader might be asked to evaluate a nursing assistant at the end of an orientation program in an extended care facility. One specific criterion which the nursing assistant is expected to achieve in relation to clients' hygiene is: "washes feet of clients who are unable to complete self-care." The nurse-leader may look at the chart of one of the clients assigned to the nursing assistant and observe that the nursing assistant has charted, "complete bed bath given." The nurse-leader may then assume that the client's feet were washed, but she cannot be sure.

The nurse-leader could inspect the client's feet. If they are clean, she may assume that the nursing assistant has washed them. This assumption would be more reasonable than the first, but again, she cannot be certain. If, however, the nurse-leader observes the nursing assistant washing the client's feet, she is then able to state without any doubt that the nursing assistant has accomplished the stated criterion.

From this example, it is obvious that obtaining data from a direct source is more accurate than using indirect sources. Why, then, are indirect sources utilized? In some cases, there is no alternative. Direct data may not be available to the evaluator—once an action is completed, it cannot be observed, and therefore, only the results and the written records are available for scrutiny. In other cases, it would be too costly and time-consuming to have an evaluator present for a long enough period of time to collect sufficient data. (One observation is usually not sufficient.) In addition, in nursing, the client's right to privacy may prevent the presence of an evaluator during interventions.

Since the goal of nursing is to promote, maintain, and restore the client's health, it seems reasonable to treat the client's response as a valid indicator of nursing care. If the client has achieved the expected goals or outcomes, then the nursing process can be said to be successful. The problem arises when the client does not achieve the outcomes; one must then ask if the nursing process has been unsuccessful. The answer may be "yes" or "no," depending on the case considered.

When the data is compared to the criteria, several possible judgments can be made: (1) the criteria have been surpassed, so that special recognition and encouragement should be given to the subject; (2) the criteria have been met, so that praise should be given; or (3) the criteria have not been met, so that assistance or direction is needed to help the subject meet the criteria. Once the judgment has been made, the evaluation process is complete.

THE EVALUATION PROCESS IN NURSING

The evaluation process is utilized in nursing as part of the larger process of quality assurance, which begins with evaluation and proceeds according to the results of the evaluation. Quality assurance is the process that ensures the delivery of health care to all persons at the optimum level of excellence, and the persistent endeavor to obtain continual improvement (Kron, 1976, p. 204). The process of quality assurance includes the entire evaluation process, and is often followed by the change process.

A quality assurance program is designed to determine the extent to which a practice achieves selected objectives (Lang, 1976, p. 5). Quality assurance programs conducted by nurses involve a process of self-regulation that demonstrates how nursing behaviors affect client progress (Beyers & Phillips, 1979, p. 117). In other words, quality assurance is one method of demonstrating accountability.

Quality assurance can be accomplished by individual nurses, groups, or organizations. Individual nurse-leaders engage in self-evaluation and often participate in group and organization evaluation; groups utilize performance appraisal and peer review to evaluate individual members; nursing audit is used to evaluate an entire group's performance; and organizations providing health care comply with the Professional Standards Review Organization (PSRO) by using the audit and the utilization review. The nurse-leader should be aware of these evaluation situations and participate in them as part of her role in quality assurance.

Self-Evaluation

Individuals often use self-evaluation in an informal, unconscious way to assess themselves. Many self-evaluations are conducted without explicit criteria, or with criteria that are unrealistic or poorly defined. Self-evaluations are, of course, of greater value when explicit, sound criteria are used. Often a job description provides realistic criteria. Personal goals, both immediate and long range, can be formulated for use in the evaluation process.

Self-evaluation is important for nurse-leaders because knowledge of self will enhance their leadership ability and potential. Self-evaluation can be an extremely accurate form of evaluation because no one knows the motivation, reasoning, and complete performance of an individual better than that individual. Before evaluating herself, the nurse-leader should review her personal philosophy of nursing as well as her immediate and long-range goals; from these, she can establish criteria.

One method of self-evaluation is to collect care plans completed for clients and, after 2 or 3 months, review them critically to see what kinds of problems were identified and what type of approaches were specified. Through such a review, the nurse-leader may be able to identify trends in her own performance. She may find that she focuses on certain problems and approaches, but overlooks others. By assessing several care plans written over a period of time, she should be able to recognize her own strengths and weaknesses in care planning. She can then set goals for herself which can serve as criteria for her next self-evaluation.

Any data collection method can be used for self-evaluation. Self-evaluation is always formative since the person involved in it is continually striving to develop and to maximize his or her potential.

Performance Appraisal

The evaluation of group members may take a variety of forms. In nursing, it is generally conducted by the nurse-leader in the form of a performance appraisal of each member.

Performance appraisals refer to evaluations of an employee conducted at regular intervals by an employer. Performance appraisals are also conducted by persons in line positions in an organization; each position in the line is evaluated by the next higher position. In nursing this means that a head nurse conducts performance appraisals of staff nurses, supervisors conduct performance appraisals of head nurses, and so on up the line.

The purpose of a performance appraisal is to encourage the development of employees who will meet the organization's objectives (Beyers & Phillips, 1979, p. 225). From the organization's point of view, productive employees are desirable and, as a result, often rewarded. On the other hand, employees who do not meet the organization's expectations are costly; in health care, they can also be dangerous. The performance appraisal provides a profile of the employee's strengths and weaknesses. The weaknesses, or performance discrepancies, can then be analyzed so that they may be eliminated, corrected, or altered to benefit both employee and organization.

Whenever a performance discrepancy is noted, certain issues must be addressed. Is the performance discrepancy a skill deficiency or a lack of knowledge? If it is either of these, continuing education programs may be an appropriate solution. The discrepancy may also result from a lack of motivation, or group members may find that not performing is more rewarding than meeting the expected criteria. In these cases, continuing education would not change performance. The activity and its consequences would probably need restructuring in order to reward the expected performance when it occurs.[2]

To conduct a productive performance appraisal, the nurse-leader should use a simple appraisal form and a format that will promote discussion between the nurse-leader evaluator and the group member being evaluated. It is essential that both persons engaging in the evaluation process have a similar understanding of the job description and of the area and scope of responsibility expected of the group member. It may be helpful if the nurse-leader begins the performance appraisal meeting by reviewing the job description and criteria with the group member being appraised. Then the nurse-leader and group member can discuss and compare what was done with the criteria.

It is usually best to focus first on the positive aspects of performance because this is more comfortable for both parties. The group member will be more receptive to comments about performance that needs improvement if the evaluator has already praised acceptable performance. All criteria need to be discussed, as well as both acceptable and unacceptable performance related to each criterion.

The discussion concludes with the development of a plan to help the group member improve performance. The time allowed for completion of this plan is the period between this appraisal and the next one—often 1 year. The plan includes methods to accomplish the goals established.

The nurse-leader evaluator writes a summary of the discussion, documenting the group member's strengths and weaknesses, goals, and plans for accomplishing the goals, and gives and overall rating of the group member. It is helpful for both parties if a working document is developed, which includes the goals set and the methods chosen for accomplishing them. Both can keep a copy of the document and can chart the progress of the group member. The data collected can then be used as evidence for the next performance appraisal (Smith & Brouwer, 1977, p. 91).

The nurse-leader doing an evaluation can prepare herself for a performance appraisal by reviewing the appraisal procedure and her observations either with her supervisor or with another nurse-leader. This will enable her to validate the method she plans to use; in addition, she may receive assistance in phrasing negative comments in such a way as to minimize defensiveness on the part of the group member. The nurse-leader

---

[2] For a checklist describing the reasons for performance discrepancies and the pertinent questions to ask, see R. F. Mager & P. Pipe. *Analyzing performance problems.* Belmont, Calif.: Lear Siegler, 1973, pp. 101–105.

must remember to evaluate performance based on her own observations and experience with the group member—not on reports from others. She should maintain open communication with her group members, and discuss incidents with them as they occur rather than wait for the performance appraisal meeting. This meeting is a time for review, a form of summative evaluation, and not a time for surprises.

When possible, the nurse-leader evaluator should have the group member rate herself before the performance appraisal meeting. The nurse-leader and group member can then compare their independent ratings. This provides a basis for discussion and usually a more objective, fair, and complete evaluation of the group member (Smith & Brouwer, 1977, p. 104).

Peer Review

Another form of group member evaluation is peer review. Peer review involves the evaluation of persons by others of equal status. Two registered nurses on the same unit with similar responsibilities may be considered peers.

Peer review differs from performance appraisal because in peer review evaluation is carried out by persons on the same level in an organization. In addition, while a self-evaluation is encouraged in performance appraisal, it is optional, whereas it is a required part of peer review.

The purpose of peer review is to have persons of the same status assist each other in recognizing the positive and negative aspects of their performance. A critical, yet empathetic, evaluation can be given by a peer. Since peers are attempting to meet the same criteria, they can make a realistic evaluation, taking into account all the facets of a job with which they are familiar.

The major problem with peer review is that some persons are afraid to give negative feedback to their peers, believing that if they do so they will receive negative feedback in return. The solution to this problem is to develop a solid base of trust among the group members. In addition, all the principles of good performance appraisals should be followed.

Peer review can be carried out in a variety of ways, and each group of nurses must decide how it can work best for them. A simple method is for the person being evaluated to evaluate her own performance according to a predetermined set of criteria and then select one or two peers to do the same. Alternatively, peers can be chosen by someone else. Finally, the person being evaluated and the peer(s) who evaluated her performance sit down together and discuss the evaluation. A plan for improvement usually emerges from the peer review. When group members, or peers, are planning and implementing their own method of peer review, their trust level should be high, so that positive benefits will result.

Nursing Audit

The third form of group member evaluation is the nursing audit. The nursing audit is used to evaluate the quality of client care, and therefore reflects the performance of a group of practitioners rather than of a single individual.

The purpose of the nursing audit is to examine nursing care that has been given to clients and verify that acceptable standards are being met. The audit is conducted after care has been provided, and is a method of accounting for outcomes achieved. Audits are usually based on the assumption that, when expected client outcomes are achieved, nursing process criteria are also met.

There are two types of nursing audits—*concurrent* and *retrospective.* The concurrent audit has also been called the *open chart* audit, because it occurs while a client is receiving care in a health care facility. The retrospective or *closed chart* audit occurs after client care has been completed, i.e., after discharge or termination of the relationship with the health care facility.

The purpose of the concurrent audit is to assess the past and present care given to a client. This type of audit can provide information to care givers that may alter a particular client's care plan. The retrospective audit also assesses care that has already been received by clients. Usually, its purpose is to assess how well the group provided care to a particular type of client. The care of clients whose charts are audited is not influenced by the outcome of a retrospective audit. However, other clients may be helped, since group members can improve the quality of care given based on the results of the audit.

Retrospective audits are less costly than concurrent audits, and usually require less time to complete. This is because records are used as the data base. Concurrent audits also use records, but in addition they often include interviews with clients and health team members. This additional data helps ensure the accuracy of a concurrent audit. When a record is unclear, the retrospective auditor must assume that the criteria has not been met, while the concurrent auditor can seek more information. The judgment of a concurrent auditor is therefore more likely to be accurate than the judgment of a retrospective auditor.

Each agency usually develops an audit form that specifies criteria of importance to that institution. Most audits are in the form of checklists and include a section for comments by the evaluator. Audit reports are ordinarily tabulated in percentages. Some agencies conclude the report with suggested activities to correct deficiencies. Discrepancies uncovered by audits may be corrected either by instituting new procedures or by instructing group members to follow existing ones. Audits also reveal what is being done well, and this provides positive reinforcement to care givers.

The nurse-leader who wishes to conduct a nursing audit should consider which type of audit best meets the needs of her group. Many organizations already conduct retrospective audits. In such a situation, the nurse-leader's responsibility is to interpret the results to her group. The retrospective audit is most useful to organizations to give an overall picture of care given to clients. The concurrent audit is most useful to those directly involved in client care. Often the motivation to improve care for a particular client is greater than the motivation to alter procedures for clients in the abstract. In other words, a group member is more likely to change his performance to benefit Mrs. Brownwin in room 746 than to benefit "thyroidectomy patients."

Professional Standards Review Organization

Organizations are responsible for the quality of care provided by all the health professionals who serve clients within their jurisdiction. To evaluate the quality of care provided in an organization, the audit and the utilization review are used. Both of these evaluation methods may be considered part of the quality assurance program known as Professional Standards Review Organization (PSRO).

In 1972, amendments to the Social Security Act mandated an evaluation system. This legislation provided for the creation of PSRO, a quality assurance program with two explicit purposes: to provide quality care to those in need and to promote cost containment (PSRO Program Manual, 1974, p. 30).

Groups of health care providers form the PSRO group, whose task is to review cases and to maintain records. PSRO initially had medical care in hospitals and nursing homes as its primary concern. In particular, the care subsidized through Medicare, Medicaid, and federally funded maternal and child health programs are within the scope of PSRO regulations.

The PSRO group is primarily responsible for determining (1) if admission to a health care facility was indicated; (2) if the duration of in-facility care was reasonable; (3) if services provided could have been more effectively and economically provided in another type of health care facility; and (4) if services provided met the PSRO criteria (Davidson, 1976, p. 88). By carrying out these four functions, the PSRO attempts to make health care providers, and physicians in particular, answerable for their decisions. The PSRO group may include all types of health team members, but since only physicians judge medical care, PSRO provides a peer review only for physicians.

PSRO has already had a great impact on health care facilities and, as the concept develops further, it is expected that the ANA *Standards of Nursing Practice* will become part of the PSRO system (Geoffrey, 1977, p. 29). It is essential that nurse-leaders become involved in PSRO to ensure that *nurses* are the ones who evaluate nursing care.

Utilization Review

The Joint Commission on Accreditation of Hospitals recommends that organizations participate in the PSRO evaluation system. In particular, organizations are expected to conduct utilization review and retrospective audits.

Utilization review is an evaluation method used within a health care facility to determine how the facility's resources are being used. The major focus of the review is occupancy. In hospitals, utilization review is done to determine if beds are occupied by clients requiring the services of an acute care facility.

The purpose of the utilization review is an attempt to decrease costs to clients by promoting discharge as soon as possible, and to make resources available to those who truly need them. Nurse-leaders often serve as evaluators for utilization review because they are in a position to make judgments about the appropriateness of care.

The retrospective audits conducted within the PSRO system encompass the nursing audit; they evaluate the independent and dependent functions of nursing as well as the care provided by all other health team members. The audit committee is most appropriately composed of several different health team members, so that all aspects of care can be judged accurately.

SUMMARY

Evaluation is the final step in many processes, but it is also a distinct process. The nurse-leader uses the three-step evaluation process very frequently. Each step in the process has been explained in detail so that the nurse-leader can use it and apply it in a variety of evaluation situations.

Performance appraisal, peer review, and nursing audit are some important types of evaluation that the nurse-leader will encounter. As nurse-leaders become more familiar with these types of evaluation and use them to improve nursing practice, nursing will become more professionalized.

REFERENCES

American Nurses' Association. *Standards of cardiovascular nursing practice.* Kansas City, 1975.

American Nurses' Association. *Standards of community health nursing practice.* Kansas City, 1974.

American Nurses' Association. *Standards of gerontological nursing practice.* Kansas City, 1976.

American Nurses' Association. *Standards of nursing practice.* Kansas City, 1973a.

American Nurses' Association. *Standards of psychiatric-mental health nursing practice.* Kansas City, 1973b.

Beyers, M., & Phillips, C. *Nursing management for patient care.* Boston: Little, Brown, 1979.

Bishop, B. E. "Quality assurance" implementation of practice standards: One mechanism. *Minnesota Nursing Accent,* 1975, *47*(1), 9–11.

Bloom, B. S., Hastings, J. T., & Madaus, G. F. *Handbook on formative and summative evaluation of student learning.* New York: McGraw-Hill, 1971.

Davidson, S. L. (Ed.). *P.S.R.O.: Utilization and audit in patient care.* St. Louis: Mosby, 1976.

Geoffrey, L. S. Professional standards review organizations. In M. E. Nicholls & V. G. Wessells (Eds.), *Nursing standards and nursing process.* Wakefield, Mass.: Contemporary Publishing, 1977.

Jucius, M. J., Deitzer, B. A., & Schlender, W. E. *Elements of managerial action.* Homewood, Ill.: Irwin, 1973.

Kron, T. *The management of patient care.* Philadelphia: Saunders, 1976.

Lang, N. M. The overview of quality assurance. In S. E. Davidson (Ed.), *P.S.R.O.: Utilization and audit in patient care.* St. Louis: Mosby, 1976.

Mager, R. F., & Pipe, P. *Analyzing performance problems.* Belmont, Calif.: Lear Siegler, 1970.

P.S.R.O. program manual. Rockville, Md.: U.S. Government Department of Health, Education, and Welfare, 1974.

Smith, H. P., & Brouwer, P. J. *Performance appraisal and human development.* Reading, Mass.: Addison-Wesley, 1977.

Thorndike, R. L., & Hagen, E. *Measurement and evaluation in psychology and education.* New York: Wiley, 1969.

ADDITIONAL READINGS

Bailit, H., Lewis, J., Hochheiser, L., & Bush, N. Assessing the quality of care. *Nursing Outlook*, 1975, *23*, 153–159.

Bloch, D. Criteria, standards, norms—Crucial terms in quality assurance. *Journal of Nursing Administration*, 1977, 7(7), 20–30.

Bloch, D. Evaluation of nursing care in terms of process and outcome: Issues in research and quality assurance. *Nursing Research*, 1975, *24*, 256–263.

Craig, J. Anecdotal records. *Canadian Nurse*, 1978, *74*(5), 25–27.

Dracup, K. Improving clinical evaluation. *Supervisor Nurse*, 1979, *10*(6), 24–27.

Haar, L. P., & Hicks, J. R. Performance appraisal: Derivation of effective assessment tools. *Journal of Nursing Administration*, 1976, *6*(7), 20–29.

Krumme, U. S. The case for criterion-referenced measurement. *Nursing Outlook*, 1975, *23*, 764–769.

Lopez, F. M. *Evaluating employee performance*. Chicago: Public Personnel Association, 1968.

Marriner, A. Evaluation of personnel. *Supervisor Nurse*, 1976, *7*(5), 36–39.

Morris, L. L., & Fitz-Gibbon, C. T. *Evaluator's handbook*. Beverly Hills: Sage, 1978.

Popham, W. J. (Ed.). *Criterion-referenced measurement: An introduction*. Englewood Cliffs, N.J.: Educational Technology Publications, 1971.

Popham, W. J., & Husek, T. R. Implications of criterion-referenced measurement. *Journal of Educational Measurement*, 1969, *6*(1), 1–9.

Ramey, I. Setting nursing standards and evaluating care. *Journal of Nursing Administration*, 1973, *3*(3), 27–35.

Ramphal, M. Peer review. *American Journal of Nursing*, 1974, *74*, 63–67.

Schwirian, P. M. Evaluating the performance of nurses: A multidimensional approach. *Nursing Research*, 1978, *27*, 347–351.

Epilogue

The analysis of the current status of the professionalization of nursing presented in Chapter 1 clearly indicates that nursing has the potential for professionalization. This potential has, as yet, not been realized. Nevertheless, the professionalization of nursing *is* possible and will occur when nurse-leaders actualize nursing leadership.

Choosing the theory and style of leadership best suited to self, follower or group, and setting will enable the nurse-leader to use the strategies of organizing, teaching-learning, decision making, changing, managing conflicts, and evaluating in a way that will produce the desired result—goal attainment. In effect, the nurse-leader develops her own fourth-level (situation-producing) theory.

If she is effective, the nurse-leader will have the ability to predict outcomes. The predicted outcomes are the goals that are established. The nurse-leader creates a situation in which goal setting and goal attainment occur.

The professionalization of nursing is one of the goals of nurse-leaders. To attain this goal, nurse-leaders need to employ systematically the strategies of nursing leadership. The strategy of organizing suggests ways of planning and setting priorities. Decision making is a much needed strategy to select from a multiplicity of options those alternatives that will indeed foster professionalization. Implementing the options that have been chosen through setting priorities and making decisions requires use of the change process. Throughout the course of professionalization, managing conflicts and employing teaching-learning strategies will be necessary. Evaluation will be inherent in all these processes.

Some specific deficits or lags in the professionalization process have been noted. What can the individual nurse-leader do to further the professionalization of nursing?

In the area of theory development, the nurse-leader can test leadership theories in her own setting. Is there a theory of leadership that promotes client health? Does one theory of leadership promote collaborative relationships within a health care team? Answering these and similar questions through research would certainly add to the development of nursing theory.

Nursing theory development will also be aided by clinically oriented research. The nursing audit may be used as a measure of quality care for research into the effectiveness of nursing interventions.

Nurses have been educated to become skilled interviewers and observers. These skills suggest a possible methodology for building a data base which could be further developed into the predictive level of theory building.

The education of nurses is currently undergoing review and critique. Conflict about entry level for professional nurses is one issue under review. Nurse-leaders in practice, research, and education must develop a comprehensive plan for the education of nurses. Evaluation of all existing educational preparation alternatives is being conducted, and decisions must be made with careful consideration of what effect the chosen option will have on individual nurses and on nursing as a whole. Nurse-leaders are needed to manage conflicts, to help their colleagues use a systematic decision-making process, and to implement planned changes.

To increase autonomy, nurse-leaders need to become increasingly accountable as well as more assertive. Peer review conducted by nurse-leaders is one way to foster the development of the four attributes (awareness, assertiveness, accountability, and advocacy) essential for effective nursing leadership.

Nurse-leaders in all settings need to become more involved in issues affecting nursing and health care. Commitment to a professional group means viewing oneself as a career member of that group, that is, an active and productive participant in the group throughout one's life. To foster professionalization, individual nurse-leaders must increase their participation in and commitment to nursing.

A strong sense of community also fosters professionalization, and this can be provided by a united professional organization. Since the American Nurses' Association (ANA) is the official professional organization of nursing, if all nurse-leaders would join ANA and work together, the organization would be strengthened immeasurably.

When change in an organization is needed, it is generally easier and more effective to bring it about from within than to have it imposed from the outside. Therefore, if nurse-leaders want ANA to change and improve, they need to join. Then, using leadership skills and working together, they can bring about necessary changes.

ANA already provides a forum for dialogue and a way for nurses to keep abreast of issues affecting nursing and health care. However, until all nurse-leaders belong to ANA, the full potential of a sense of community will not be achieved.

Nurse-leaders are needed to further the professionalization of nursing. Their ability to attain this goal is unquestionable; willingness is all that is required. The purpose of this book about nursing leadership and its components and strategies has been to develop nurse-leaders who are both able and willing to assist nursing in its development toward full professionalization. As nurses become truly effective leaders, it will become clear to them that leadership is indeed the key to the professionalization of nursing.

Index